Copyright © 2016 by Trivium Test Prep

ALL RIGHTS RESERVED. By purchase of this book, you have been licensed one copy for personal use only. No part of this work may be reproduced, redistributed, or used in any form or by any means without prior written permission of the publisher and copyright owner.

Trivium Test Prep is not affiliated with or endorsed by any testing organization and does not own or claim ownership of any trademarks, specifically for the CHPN (Certified Hospice and Palliative Nurse) exam. All test names (and their acronyms) are trademarks of their respective owners. This study guide is for general information and does not claim endorsement by any third party.

TABLE OF CONTENTS

I. PATIENT CARE

Identifying and Responding to the Indicators of Imminent Death	7
Identifying Specific Patterns of the Progression	11
Enteral and Parenteral Nutrition	29
Delirium and Dementia	33
Endocrine Disorders	37

II. PAIN MANAGEMENT

Introduction to the Nursing Process	41
A Comprehensive Pain Assessment	45
Pharmacological Interventions	49
Dosage Equivalents	53
Administering Adjuvant Medications	57
Interactions and Side Effects	71
Non-Pharmacological Interventions	75

III. SYMPTOM MANAGEMENT

Neurological Symptoms	81
Cardiovascular Symptoms	93
Respiratory Symptoms	97

Gastrointestinal Symptoms - - - - - - 101

Genitourinary Symptoms - - - - - - 109

Musculoskeletal Symptoms - - - - - - 113

Skin and Mucous Membrane Symptoms - - - - 119

Psychosocial, Spiritual and Emotional Issues - - - 123

Nutritional and Metabolic Symptoms - - - - - 139

Immune and Lymphatic Symptoms - - - - - 153

Mental Status Changes - - - - - - - 157

IV. CARE OF THE PATIENT AND FAMILY

Identifying Goals and Outcomes - - - - - 167

Developing a Plan and Evaluating Progress - - - - 171

Resource Management - - - - - - - 175

Assessing Safety and Responding to Environmental Risks - 179

Psychosocial, Spiritual and Cultural Issues - - - - 185

V. EDUCATION AND ADVOCACY

Caregiver Support - - - - - - - - 193

Education - - - - - - - - - 197

Advocacy - - - - - - - - - 211

VI. INTERDISCIPLINARY AND COLLABORATIVE PRACTICE

Supervision and Delegation - - - - - - 217

Collaboration - - - - - - - - 221

VII. PROFESSIONAL ISSUES

Practice Issues - - - - - - - - 227

Incorporating Guidelines into Practice - - - - 235

Incorporating Legal Regulations into Practice - - - 239

Professional Development - - - - - - 249

VIII. PRACTICE QUESTIONS - - - - - 253

Answer Key - - - - - - - - 283

Exclusive Trivium Test Tips - - - - - 285

CERTIFIED HOSPICE AND PALLIATIVE NURSE (CHPN)

Hospice and palliative nurses work as part of interdisciplinary teams caring for patients with life-limiting illnesses and their families. Settings offer nursing support twenty-four hours a day, symptom and pain management, and support to the family. Support includes caring for not only physical but also psychosocial, emotional, and spiritual needs of patients. In order to provide the highest level of hospice and palliative care, the advanced practice nurse, nurse, licensed practical/vocational nurse, pediatric nurse, nursing assistant and administrator must function as a team.

I. PATIENT CARE

Dying clients have quite different needs than others. Patients die as the result of one of three patterns. They die from a steady decline over a relatively brief period, such as clients affected with cancer. They decline over a long period, such as in the case of chronic illness and events like cerebrovascular disease. Lastly, clients die as the result of an acute episode or exacerbation of an existing disease, such a sudden acute myocardial infarction or death from heart failure. It is less complicated and challenging to determine life expectancy and the time of death among those who have steady decline over a relatively brief period as occurs among clients affected with cancer, than it is among those who have a chronic disorder of prolonged duration.

When a client is potentially dying, they should be given complete information and the opportunity to discuss their care goals and make decisions about many things including financial issues, family issues, final wishes and whether or not to undergo medical treatments or elect to choose palliative and hospice care.

IDENTIFYING AND RESPONDING TO THE INDICATORS OF IMMINENT DEATH

Like so many biological events, death is a process. The perideath experience consists of the preparation for death, the death itself, and the third phase, which is after death. The nurses play an important role in all three of these phases of perideath.

Some of the signs and symptoms that occur during phase one, the preparation for death, include:

- Bodily coolness
- Excessive sleeping
- Decreases of food and fluids
- Incontinence
- Congestion

- Changes in breathing patterns, including Cheyne-Stokes respirations
- Disorientation
- Restlessness
- Withdrawal
- Vision-like experiences
- Letting go
- Saying goodbye

IDENTIFYING SPECIFIC PATTERNS OF THE PROGRESSION

Hematological, Oncologic and Paraneoplastic Disorders

Hypercalcemia

Hypercalcemia is high levels of calcium in the blood.

Risk Factors

Oncology patients are at risk particularly when they are affected with primary cancer of, or metastasis to, the bone, lung cancer, breast cancer, and cancers of the blood like multiple myeloma. Some of the specific pathophysiological changes, in addition to hypercalcemia and low serum phosphate, include renal calculi, demineralization of the bone, hypokalemia and metabolic acidosis.

Signs and Symptoms

Of the many signs and symptoms, bone pain, muscular weakness, anorexia, nausea, vomiting, abdominal pain, cardiac arrhythmias, paresthesia, depression, weight loss and psychosis can occur.

Treatment

Patients who are symptomatic with signs of hypercalcemia may require extensive intravenous fluid replacement, large doses of vitamins A and D, loop diuretics, decreased calcium intake, an increased fluid intake of 2 liters or more per day, and medications, such as zoledronate, alendronate or pamidronate. A surgical partial or complete removal of the parathyroid glands may also be required as indicated.

Safety is a primary concern since pathological bone fractures can occur.

Related Nursing Diagnoses

- At risk for pathological fractures r/t bone decalcification
- Pain r/t skeletal bone decalcification
- Dehydration r/t hypercalcemia
- At risk for kidney failure r/t hypercalcemia

Shock

Simply stated, shock is a condition where the body tissue is not sufficiently perfused. The oxygen and nutritional demands exceed the amount of oxygen and nutrients available. The five types of shock are anaphylactic shock, septic shock, neurogenic shock, carcinogenic shock, and hypovolemic shock. All types of shock are life threatening.

- Anaphylactic shock: This type of shock is an allergic response.

- Septic shock: Septic shock is a systemic, multisystem response to an infection. It is characterized by a high incidence of morbidity and mortality.

- Neurogenic shock: This form of shock results when damage to the central nervous system occurs. It results in hypotension and bradycardia because of decreased vascular resistance.

- Cardiogenic shock: This form of shock occurs when the ventricles of the heart are not functioning properly; this malfunction leads to inadequate circulation.

- Hypovolemic shock: The most common type of shock. There is insufficient circulatory volume.

Hypovolemic Shock and Hemorrhage

Risk Factors

Risk factors include hemorrhage, including post-operative hemorrhage after cancer surgery, severe diarrhea and vomiting, and profound dehydration.

Signs and Symptoms

The signs and symptoms vary according to the stage of the hypovolemic shock.

- Initial Stage: Hypoxia occurs as the result of hypoperfusion.

- Compensatory Stage: Compensatory mechanisms such as hyperventilation (to raise PH and decrease carbon dioxide levels), decreased cardiac output (vasodilation), tachycardia (norepinephrine and epinephrine release), and diminished urinary output (anti-diuretic hormone release to protect the kidneys with vasopression) occur.

- Progressive Stage: Metabolic acidosis, increased blood viscosity and impaired microcirculation severely compromise the perfusion of all vital organs (multisystem failure.)

- Refractory or Irreversible Stage: Vital organs have failed; and death is imminent.

Treatment

Ongoing assessments, the immediate correction of the cause (bleeding, dehydration) and the replacement of blood and fluid volume are necessary to preserve life. Multiple intravenous catheters are placed and fluids like lactated ringers, blood, blood components and plasma expanders are used, as indicated.

Nurses must monitor urinary output, vital signs, central venous pressure and arterial blood gases among other things. The client should be placed in the Trendelenberg position, unless contraindicated, to promote venous return.

Related Nursing Diagnoses

- Fear and anxiety r/t a serious threat to health status
- Ineffective tissue perfusion r/t hypovolemic shock
- At risk for injury and death r/t multiple organ failure
- Deficient fluid volume r/t hemorrhage and third spacing

Septic Shock

Septic shock is a systemic, multisystem response to an infection. It is characterized by a high incidence of morbidity and mortality.

Risk Factors

Some of the factors that place clients at risk for septic shock include a surgical or invasive procedure infection, immunocompromise, leukemia, and lymphoma, all of which can affect oncology clients.

Some of the most common pathogens that lead to sepsis and septic shock are gram-negative bacteria, such as Escherichia coli (E. coli) and pseudomonas aeruginosa, gram-positive bacteria like staphylococcus aureus and streptococcus pneumonia, and other microorganisms like a virus, fungus and parasites.

Signs and Symptoms

Several pathophysiological changes like massive vasodilation, the formation of microemboli, cardiac depression, and the abnormal distribution of intravascular fluid occur.

The early stage is marked with hypotension, flushed, warm skin, a widened pulse pressure, massive vasodilation and decreased systemic vascular resistance, tachycardia, hyperventilation, metabolic acidosis, respiratory alkalosis, adventitious breath sounds like crackles, hypoxia, pulmonary edema, confusion, lethargy and other symptoms of hypoxia occur. Later, as cardiac output dramatically decreases, peripheral vasoconstriction and life threatening hypoxia affects multiple bodily systems.

Prevention

Some of the ways that infections, bacteremia, sepsis and septic shock can be prevented are to minimize the use of invasive procedures and treatments to the greatest extent possible. All invasive procedures, like surgery, and all invasive treatments, like central lines, intravenous lines, and urinary catheters, place patients at risk for an infection.

Treatment

Fluids are administered to restore fluid that has left the vascular spaces and to correct for the peripheral vasodilation. Other treatments can include mechanical ventilation, oxygen supplementation, possible dialysis, and medications including antibiotics for the infection, medications to increase the blood pressure and ongoing hemodynamic monitoring.

Nurses must adhere to standard precautions, special precautions, medical and surgical asepsis techniques and hand washing protocols as well as closely monitor and assess patients for any sign of infection, particularly when they are immunocompromised with an immunosuppressive disease, chemotherapy and/or the use of steroidal medications.

Related Nursing Diagnoses

- Altered mental status r/t hypoxia
- At risk death r/t sepsis and septic shock
- Ineffective tissue perfusion r/t decreased systemic vascular resistance
- Impaired hemodynamic regulation r/t sepsis and septic shock

Tumor Lysis Syndrome

Tumor lysis syndrome is a group of metabolic complications that can occur as the result of cancer treatments. This oncological emergency occurs with the presence of massive tumor that releases large amounts of potassium, nucleic acids and phosphate into the patient's systematic circulation.

Risk Factors

Risk factors for tumor lysis syndrome include large tumors, tumors with rapid cell division and growth, hematologic cancers like acute leukemia, aggressive tumors, and lymphoma.

Patients with non-Hodgkin's lymphoma, adult lymphoblastic leukemia, acute lymphoid leukemia, lymphomas such as Burkett's lymphoma, large B-cell lymphoma, monoblastic acute myeloid leukemia, and acute monoblastic leukemia, are at risk. Other risk factors include chemotherapy in its first cycle, renal impairment, preexisting dehydration and preexisting hyperuricemia.

Symptoms of tumor lysis syndrome can occur within seventy-two hours after the initiation of cytotoxic therapy.

Signs and Symptoms

Abdominal pain and distension, edema, lethargy, sudden death, syncope, cardiac dysrhythmias, congestive heart failure, fluid overload, hyperkalemia (muscular weakness), hypocalcaemia (vomiting, anorexia, seizures, cramps, spasms, and altered mental status), and urinary symptoms, such as hematuria, flank pain, oliguria and dysuria, can occur.

Prevention

Patients at risk should receive aggressive IV hydration. The ultimate goal of this type of prevention is to improve renal function and glomerular filtration and to increase the urine output, which can minimize the chance of uric acid and/or calcium phosphate precipitation in the tubules.

Treatment

The management of tumor lysis includes immediate supportive care in terms of IV hydration and the correction of metabolic alterations to preserve life. Dialysis is necessary in extreme cases of hyperkalemia and/or renal failure. Dietary restrictions in terms of potassium, phosphorus and /or uric acid are recommended, as well as medications like allopurinol and rasburicase.

Nurses must closely assess clients for the signs and symptoms of tumor lysis, particularly those at risk and those in the beginning stages of chemotherapy.

Related Nursing Diagnoses

- Impaired renal function r/t tumor lysis
- At risk for injury r/t tumor lysis
- Anxiety r/t life threatening event

Neurological Disorders

Increased Intracranial Pressure

Normal intracranial pressure (ICP) is from 5 to 15 mmHg. Increased ICP occurs when the volume of the cranial cavity increases, such as occurs with the presence of a cerebral tumor and hydrocephalus. Brain herniation occurs when intracranial pressure increases without successful treatment.

Risk Factors

In addition to a brain tumor and hydrocephalus, other risk factors include head trauma, a cerebral infarction, a subdural or epidural hematoma, and infections.

Signs and Symptoms

Some of the commonly occurring signs and symptoms include Cushing's reflex and Cheyne-Stokes respirations. Cushing's reflex indicates that brainstem ischemia is present; it is marked with bradycardia, a widening pulse pressure and hypertension.

Treatment

Some of the medications that are used include intravenous osmotic diuretics, like mannitol, to remove fluid, corticosteroids to reduce edema, and anticonvulsant medications to prevent seizures. A barbiturate coma is sometimes necessary to lower the metabolic demands of the brain and to prevent further brain damage. Additionally, artificial ventilation is often necessary and surgical interventions are sometimes necessary to eliminate the cause of the ICP if the client chooses these intervention.

Ongoing neurological assessments are indicated.

Related Nursing Diagnoses

- At risk for brain herniation r/t increased intracranial pressure
- At risk for seizures r/t increased intracranial pressure
- Impaired cognitive functioning r/t increased intracranial pressure

Spinal Cord Compression

Spinal cord compression is an emergency that can lead to irreversible paraplegia.

Risk Factors

Risk factors for spinal cord compression are pressure from tumors that are expanding in terms of size, such as tumors of the lung, prostate or breast(s.) It is also associated with lymphoma and metastatic disease.

Signs and Symptoms

Back pain, numbness, paresthesia, weakness, coldness of the leg, leg pain, bladder and bowel dysfunction, and paralysis can occur.

Treatment

Treatment for spinal cord compression can be rendered with either radiation or a surgical intervention. Close monitoring and ongoing neurological assessments are indicated.

Related Nursing Diagnoses

- At risk for injury r/t numbness and paresthesia of the legs
- Pain r/t spinal cord compression
- At risk for paralysis r/t spinal cord compression

Cardiac Disorders

<u>Superior Vena Cava Syndrome</u>

Superior vena cava syndrome decreases the amount of blood that can return to the heart because the vena cava is compressed and blood backs up into the venous system. It typically occurs as the result of a tumor, which blocks the flow of blood, but it can also result from a thrombus around a subclavian arterial catheter.

Risk Factors

The most common risk factor is a tumor in the mediastinum between the lungs, under the breastbone.

Signs and Symptoms

The signs and symptoms of superior vena cava syndrome tend to develop over time. The first symptoms that appear are facial, periorbital and/or arm edema. Respiratory distress, tachypnea, altered consciousness, dyspnea, cyanosis and neurological deficits, increased venous pressure, venous stasis and engorgement of veins occur as it progresses.

Treatment

When faced with this emergency, it is essential to provide the patient with respiratory support along with oxygen. Preparations should be made for a tracheotomy. Monitor the patient's vital signs; corticosteroids, such as dexamethasone, are needed to reduce edema. Anticoagulant, or antifibrinolytic, medications are necessary if the problem is related to a clot. A safe environment including precautions for seizures should be provided, and once the emergency is under control the patient may need to receive chemotherapy or radiation for a reduction in size of the tumor.

Related Nursing Diagnoses

- Respiratory distress r/t superior vena cava syndrome
- At risk for diminished level consciousness r/t hypoxia
- Impaired cardiac output r/t superior vena cava syndrome
- Impaired respiratory functioning r/t superior vena cava syndrome

<u>Cardiac Tamponade</u>

This life-threatening emergency occurs when the pericardial sac rapidly collects fluid. This collection of fluid interferes with ventricular filling and pumping, and compression of the heart.

Risk Factors

Oncology clients are at risk when affected with breast, lung or other cancers invading the pericardial sac and high dosage levels of radiation. Other risk factors include an accidental puncture of the chest cavity and hypothyroidism.

Signs and Symptoms

Signs and symptoms of cardiac tamponade include low urine output, tachycardia, mottled, cool skin, hypotension, a narrowed pulse pressure, weak peripheral pulses, muffled heart sounds, a decreased level of consciousness, jugular vein distension and high central venous pressure.

Treatment

Fluid in the pericardial sac is drained by pericardiocentesis. There are occasions when a portion or the entire pericardial sac is removed in order to relieve pressure on the patient's heart. Oxygen, intravenous fluids and medications are necessary to increase the client's blood pressure and the underlying cause is corrected immediately after the client is stabilized.

Cardiac tamponade requires that the nurse closely monitor and assess the client and render treatments in a timely manner.

Related Nursing Diagnoses

- At risk for death r/t impaired cardiac output
- Impaired cardiac output r/t hypotension
- Anxiety r/t a life threatening event

Pulmonary Disorders

Chronic Obstructive Pulmonary Disease (COPD)

Chronic obstructive pulmonary disease (COPD) is a chronic, progressive pulmonary disorder characterized by obstructed airflow, inflammation, narrowing and scarring of peripheral airways, closure of the small airways, parenchymal and alveoli lung cell damage, loss of lung elasticity, and varying degrees of impaired gas exchange.

Risk Factors

The risk factors associated with COPD include cigarette smoking and second hand smoke. It is most common among middle age and older adults, African Americans and the male sex.

Signs and Symptoms

Some of the signs and symptoms included a decrease in FEV1, as the result of hypoxemia and hypercapnia, dyspnea, shortness of breath, pallor, a productive cough, pulmonary hypertension, agitation, tachypnea, wheezing, fatigue, and a decreased level of consciousness.

Treatment

Depending on the client's level of oxygenation, COPD is treated with bronchodilators, respiratory nebulizer treatments, oxygen and, at times, mechanical ventilation.

Related Nursing Diagnoses

- Activity intolerance r/t an oxygen demand that is greater than the oxygen supply
- Anxiety r/t shortness of breath and dyspnea
- Death anxiety r/t a feeling of suffocation

Pneumonitis

Pneumonitis is the inflammation of lung tissue.

Risk Factors

Chemotherapy drugs and radiation can cause pneumonitis and the combination of the two further increases the risk.

Signs and Symptoms

There are several signs and symptoms of pneumonitis, and the most common is shortness of breath. Other signs and symptoms include a cough, shortness of breath, fatigue, anorexia, and weight loss.

Treatment

Avoiding chemicals that the patient is hypersensitive to is an obvious treatment for pneumonitis. In more severe cases, treatment can include antibiotics for a bacterial infection, corticosteroids, such as prednisone, to reduce the inflammation, and oxygen therapy can be used if the patient is having difficulties breathing. If left untreated, it can develop into chronic pneumonitis.

Nurses must assess clients for the warning signs and symptoms of pneumonitis, particularly those clients at risk for it.

Related Nursing Diagnoses

- Alteration of respiratory status r/t pneumonitis
- Dyspnea r/t pneumonitis

Respiratory Secretions at the End of Life

At the end of life, respiratory noises occur because of air passing through airways that have secretions. These upper airway noises signal that the end of life is likely to occur within forty-eight hours.

Treatment

These noises can be somewhat disturbing to the client's family members and loved ones, so it is important to educate them about what the noises are and what causes them. In many cases, these noises can be diminished or eliminated by repositioning the client.

Related Nursing Diagnoses

- Significant other anxiety r/t secretions at the end of life
- Alteration of respiratory function r/t secretions at the end of life

Renal and Urinary Tract Disorders

Urinary Tract Infections

E. coli is the most commonly offending pathogen associated with urinary tract infections among females. Females are at greater risk for UTIs than males because of their anatomical differences in terms of a shorter urethra and the structural proximity of the urethra to the rectum, vaginal canal, and coital secretions. Klebsiella, proteus and staphylococcus, in addition to E. coli, can also cause urinary tract infections. Males typically present with a urinary tract infections secondary to some obstructive process like hypertrophy of the prostate gland.

Risk Factors

One of the most common causes of a urinary tract infection is an indwelling urinary catheter. For this reason, the use of these urinary catheters should be restricted to only those clients who absolutely need them and, then, when used, they should remain in place for the briefest period possible.

Signs and Symptoms

The client assessment will reveal dysuria, burning on urination, frequency, urgency, nocturia, pain and discomfort in the suprapubic area and gross or microscopic hematuria.

Treatment

Urinary tract infections are treated with a combination of antibiotics and analgesia when indicated. When left untreated, they can lead to renal failure. Nurses should encourage a daily fluid intake of 3 liters per day and discourage the ingestion of bladder irritants such as alcohol, cola soft drinks, caffeine and aspartame. The nurse should also educate the client about ways to prevent these infections including voiding immediately after coitus, proper perineal care, wiping from the front to the back, and wearing only cotton underwear.

Preventing Catheter-Associated Urinary Tract Infections (CAUTI)

Catheter-associated urinary tract infections (CAUTI) are a major concern in healthcare. All invasive procedures and treatments, such as catheters, place patients at risk for infection. These infections can affect any area of the urinary system, including the bladder, ureters, urethra, and kidney.

Preventative measures for catheter-associated urinary tract infections include:

- Inserting and using urinary catheters only when necessary
- The removal of the catheter as soon as possible
- The insertion, care and maintenance of the catheter by only those that are competent to do
- Maintaining strict aseptic technique
- The use of sterile supplies and equipment
- Maintaining unobstructed urinary flow
- Hand washing
- Maintaining a closed urinary drainage system without disconnecting the catheter from tubing or the tubing from the drainage bag
- Securing the catheter to the leg to prevent pulling on the catheter
- Avoiding any kinking or twisting of the catheter
- Always keeping the catheter and bag lower than the level of the bladder to prevent any urinary backflow
- Keep the bag lower than the bladder to prevent urine from back flowing to the bladder
- Emptying the collection bag frequently and not touching the drainage spout with anything

Some alternatives, like a portable ultrasound devices to assess urine volume and antimicrobial-impregnated catheters, such as silver-alloy coated catheters, may reduce the risk for catheter-associated urinary tract infections by eliminating the need for catheterization and preventing infection, respectively. Additionally, external condom catheters may be necessary for male patients and intermittent catheterization, rather than an indwelling catheter should be considered.

Related Nursing Diagnoses

- Acute pain r/t urinary tract infection
- Impaired urinary elimination r/t urinary tract infection

Nephropathy

Diabetic nephropathy, a renal glomerular disorder, is a preventable complication of diabetes that is the leading cause of chronic renal failure in our nation.

The pathological changes that occur as the result of diabetic nephropathy include the sclerosis of the glomeruli, a thickening of the glomerular membrane, and mesangial expansion. These pathophysiological changes lead to decreased glomerular filtration rates and glomerular hypertension.

Risk Factors

The primary risk factor is uncontrolled diabetes.

Signs and Symptoms

This disorder may remain asymptomatic until the client develops renal failure or nephritic syndrome. The diagnosis of this disorder is based on the presence of urinary albumin. A ratio > 30 mg/g or an albumin excretion of 30 to 300 mg/24 h suggests the early stage of diabetic nephropathy. Advanced diabetic nephropathy is signaled with a positive urine dipstick for protein. This positive dipstick indicates that the albumin excretion is more than 300 mg/day.

Treatment

Treatment aims to control the client's blood pressure and the client's control of their blood glucose. An ACE inhibitor, an angiotensin II receptor blocker, or a combination of both may be necessary to control the client's hypertension.

Careful monitoring of the client's blood pressure and blood glucose levels are essential.

Related Nursing Diagnoses

- At risk for renal failure r/t nephropathy
- At risk for cardiac and cerebrovascular events r/t nephropathy

Gastrointestinal and Hepatic Disorders

Cancer of the Stomach

Gastric cancer is a leading cause of cancer morbidity and mortality. The diffuse form of this adenocarcinoma has a higher mortality rate than the intestinal form. Metastasis most often affects the pancreas, spleen, liver, esophagus, lungs, bones and adjacent lymph nodes.

Risk Factors

Some of the risk factors associated with cancer of the stomach include cigarette smoking, H. pylori gastritis, a diet high in sodium and/or nitrates, a diet that is low in fresh vegetables and fruits, and possibly genetics.

Signs and Symptoms

Dyspepsia, nausea, often drastic weight loss, cachexia, bowel obstruction, epigastric pain, weakness and discomfort are common signs and symptoms.

Treatment

A combination of radiation and surgery with a Billroth I or Billroth II gastric resection is the typical treatment. These surgical procedures can lead to vitamin B12 deficiencies, dumping syndrome, malabsorption and duodenal reflux.

Nurse must monitor clients for complications like bowel obstructions and address any nutritional challenges.

Related Nursing Diagnoses

- Pain r/t cancer of the stomach and metastasis
- Impaired nutrition r/t malabsorption

Cancer of the Esophagus

This form of cancer also has a high morbidity and mortality rate because it is typically not diagnosed until the entire esophagus is affected.

Risk Factors

Some of the risk factors include obesity, alcohol abuse, smoking, reflux disorders and foods contaminated with nitrosamines. Esophageal cancer most often affects the male sex and those of African-American descent.

Signs and Symptoms

Some of the signs and symptoms are heartburn, odynophagia (substernal chest pain,) weight loss, dysphagia, foul breath, regurgitation and anorexia. Complications include metastasis, dysphagia, obstruction, pulmonary complications and weight loss. Post surgical complications include bleeding, infection, and leakage of the anastomosis.

Treatment

Esophageal cancer is typically treated with a combination of surgery (total or subtotal esophagectomy or an esophagogastrostomy with gastric pull through), chemotherapy and radiation.

Parenteral or enteral nutrition, which are discussed below, are often needed to sustain the client, particularly after surgery, in order to maintain good nutrition and optimal healing.

The client should be assessed for any complications and treated for pain associated with this disorder.

Related Nursing Diagnoses

- Potential airway obstruction r/t dysphagia
- Pain r/t surgery

Colorectal Cancer

Colorectal cancer is a common form of cancer found in developed nations. It can metastasize to other sites and it can lead to massive gastrointestinal bleeding and death.

Risk Factors

Colorectal cancer is associated with obesity, those over 60 years of age, cigarette smoking, ulcerative colitis, polyps, genetics, environmental factors, Crohn's disease, a diet poor in fiber and high in terms of refined fats, proteins and/or carbohydrates, estrogen and progesterone supplementation, and the long term use of NSAIDs.

Signs and Symptoms

Colon cancer, often asymptomatic, can present with bowel obstruction, abdominal pain, red rectal bleeding, weight loss, anorexia, malaise, bloating, black tarry stools, diarrhea and constipation.

Treatment

The treatment of colon cancer can include surgery (colon resection, colostomy) chemotherapy, and radiation, depending on the location and severity as well as the client's choices.

Related Nursing Diagnoses

- Anxiety r/t surgery
- Pain r/t the cancer and its signs/symptoms
- Altered body image r/t colostomy

Cancer of the Pancreas

Most pancreatic cancers form in the head of the pancreas. This form of cancer rapidly progresses and death usually occurs from one to three years after diagnosis.

Risk Factors

Males, cigarette smokers, and those over 60 years of age are at risk. It also appears that cancer of the pancreas could be genetic.

The signs and symptoms include dull epigastric pain, jaundice, weight loss, anorexia and ascites. Some of the complications associated with pancreatic cancer are malnutrition, pain and eventual death.

Treatment

A pancreatoduodenectomy may be necessary when this cancer is diagnosed in the early stages, but most often, it is diagnosed in its later stages so the treatment typically consists of palliative radiation and chemotherapy for the relief of some of the symptoms.

Related Nursing Diagnoses

- Anticipatory grieving r/t terminal illness
- Death anxiety r/t pancreatic cancer

Cancer of the Liver

Most cases of cancer of the liver are the result of metastasis from another site, although some cases can also be a primary site. Death usually occurs within 6 or 8 weeks after diagnosis when left untreated.

Risk Factors

The risk factors associated with primary site liver cancer include alcohol-related and hepatitis B and/or C-related liver disease. Liver cancer, as a secondary cancer site, occurs most often with cancer of the lung, kidney, breast, and other gastrointestinal sites.

Signs and Symptoms

Liver cancer can be asymptomatic or manifested with the typical signs and symptoms of liver disease and liver failure such as anorexia, weakness, fatigue, abdominal pain, and weight loss.

Treatment

Chemotherapy with high doses of fluorodeoxyuridine and 5-fluorouracil is necessary when a liver resection is not a treatment option. This chemotherapy can be administered intravenously or directly into the liver using a hepatic arterial infusion.

Related Nursing Diagnoses

- Ineffective family coping r/t terminal disease with a rapid progression
- Alteration of nutritional status r/t anorexia

ENTERAL AND PARENTERAL NUTRITION

Some at the end of life choose to have enteral or parenteral nutrition and others elect to forgo this form of nutrition. These artificial forms of nutrition, when used, are most often necessary for clients with severe gastrointestinal disorders such as cancer and malabsorption.

Enteral nutrition delivers nourishment and nutrients directly into the gastrointestinal tract with a tube feeding like a nasogastric tube feeding or a gastrostomy tube feeding. Nasogastric tube feedings are the preferred method except when the client is affected with a swallowing disorder, impaired gag reflex and/or a disorder of the esophageal sphincter that could potentially lead to reflux. When long term enteral feeding is necessary, a percutaneous endoscopic gastrostomy (PEG) tube is endoscopically introduced into the stomach and through the abdominal wall with the use of a local anesthetic.

Enteral nutrition, similar to parenteral nutrition, consists of essential nutrients and many different solutions that vary in terms of their osmolality, calories and proportions of fat, carbohydrates and protein. Solutions are selected based on the client's needs. These feedings can be delivered on a continuous basis, intermittently or as a bolus.

Unlike enteral nutrition, parenteral nutrition is delivered intravenously. This method is preferred when the client needs, and chooses to, have nutritional support for more than one week. Complications of parenteral nutrition include bacterial contamination, aspiration, diarrhea (particularly when a high caloric density formula is used) and regurgitation.

Although this form of nutrition can be delivered through a peripheral vein, it is most often delivered with a central venous catheter and a port. Scrupulous sterile dressing changes must be done in order to prevent infection, which is a commonly occurring complication of parenteral nutrition. Other complications are air embolus, infection, and metabolic disturbances like glucose intolerance.

General Debility: Failure to Thrive and Malabsorption

People who fail to thrive do not utilize the calories they needed to gain and maintain weight. Children are most affected with this disorder. Permanent physical and mental damage occurs.

Risk Factors

Some of the risk factors include poverty and neglect, gastrointestinal problems like chronic diarrhea, chronic liver disease, gastroesophageal reflux disease (GERD), cystic fibrosis and celiac disease, chronic illnesses like cancer and tuberculosis, infections, and metabolic disorders that limit the client's ability to break down foods into energy effectively.

Signs and Symptoms

Some symptoms of failure to thrive include irritability, the avoidance of eye contact, loss of interest, and not reaching developmental milestones.

Treatment

Treatments vary according to the cause and the severity of this disorder. For example, if the failure to thrive is the result of a chronic illness like chronic liver disease, a gastroenterologist should treat the disease. When this disorder is the result of caregiver neglect, for example, a social worker, psychologist or another mental health professional should be consulted. In severe cases, the patient may require tube feeding.

Related Nursing Diagnoses

- Failure to thrive r/t depression, apathy and/or fatigue
- Inadequate nutrition r/t failure to thrive

Malabsorption

If a disorder interferes with the digestion of food or if it interferes directly with the absorption of nutrients, malabsorption occurs.

Risk Factors

The risk factors associated with malabsorption include the presence of lactase deficiency, increased digestive acid production, decreased digestive enzyme production, decreased bile, some medications like cholestyramine, tetracycline, and colchicine, infections, alcohol use, and disorders, such as celiac disease, Chron's disease, intestinal wall lymphoma and an inadequate supply of blood to the small intestine.

Signs and Symptoms

The most common symptom is chronic diarrhea. Steatorrhea results from the inadequate absorption of fats in the digestive tract. Explosive diarrhea, abdominal bloating and flatulence can all result from the inadequate absorption of sugars.

Deficiencies of nutrients, minerals, fats, proteins, and sugars can be result from malabsorption. Weight loss, edema, dry skin, hair loss, anemia, fatigue and weakness can occur.

Treatment

The signs and symptoms of malabsorption, like diarrhea, are treated alongside any underlying disorder. When nutritional status is severely compromised, enteral and parenteral nutrition, as discussed above, is initiated.

Related Nursing Diagnoses

- Imbalanced nutrition: less than body requirements r/t inability of the body to absorb necessary nutrients
- Risk for deficient fluid volume r/e diarrhea

DELIRIUM AND DEMENTIA

Delirium

Delirium is a serious disturbance to a patient's mental abilities. The patient will suffer a decreased awareness of their surroundings and confusion. Delirium comes on suddenly, usually within a few hours or over a few days. It is common at the end of life for a client to experience delirium.

Risk Factors

Delirium can be caused by cerebral tumors, severe or chronic mental illness, medications, infections, surgery, drug/alcohol abuse, an accumulation of toxins as the result of liver or renal failure, metabolic and electrolyte imbalances.

Signs and Symptoms

Clients with delirium oftentimes experience bouts of delirium interspersed with periods of lucidity. The primary symptoms of delirium include reduced awareness of the environment and environmental stimuli, cognitive impairment and behavioral changes, such as extreme fear, anxiety, depression, anger, changes in sleep habits, restlessness, agitation, irritability, combative behavior, and hallucinations.

The only prevention for delirium is to avoid the risk factors that can cause an episode to occur. For hospitalized patients, these risk factors can include loud noises, poor lighting, a lack of natural light, invasive procedures and frequent room changes. There are certain things that the nurses, and other members of the healthcare team, can do to prevent the possibility of an episode of delirium from triggering, including:

- Pain management
- Natural forms of sleep and anxiety management
- Prevention of sleep interruptions
- Adequate fluids

When the patient's level of health prior to the delirium is good, they are likely to recover fully. Delirium among the seriously ill can result in permanent alterations of the patient's thinking and/or functioning levels.

Treatment

The treatment includes the elimination of the cause or trigger of the delirium and supportive care to prevent complications from occurring. This includes protecting the airway, providing the patient with sufficient fluids and nutrition, pain management, and keeping the environment familiar and patient-oriented. Medications can be helpful for treating some of the symptoms, like hallucination, severe agitation, confusion, fear or paranoia.

At the end of life, the cause of delirium is often irreversible; therefore, managing the symptoms is the ultimate goal of treatment. Client's family members and loved ones are often encouraged to speak to the client even if they are unconscious, because research has shown that the client may be able to understand these conversations, and it is helpful for the family and loved ones to be able to say anything they may feel they were unable to say previously.

Related Nursing Diagnoses

- Acute confusion r/t delirium
- At risk for injury r/t delirium
- Adult failure to thrive r/t delirium
- Disturbed thought processes and impaired memory r/t delirium

Dementia

Dementia is not considered a specific disease, but rather a group of symptoms that affect a patient's thinking and their social abilities so severely that they interfere with the patient's everyday life and functioning. Unlike delirium, which can be treated and reversed, most cases of dementia are not reversible. Alzheimer's syndrome is the number one cause of progressive dementia.

Signs and Symptoms

The signs and symptoms of dementia vary depending on the actual cause of the dementia. Some examples include hallucination, delusions, memory loss, agitation, paranoia, personality changes and problems performing usual activities. Nurses must modify care and communication as based on the client's symptoms.

Treatment

The exact prevention of dementia is not known, but it has been shown that some things can lessen the symptoms and slow down the progression of this disorder. Some recommendations for the client include keeping an active mind, remaining physically and socially active, decreasing the blood pressure and healthy eating. Some helpful medications include memantine and cholinesterase inhibitors.

Related Nursing Diagnoses

- At risk for injury r/t dementia
- Adult failure to thrive r/t dementia
- Chronic confusion r/t dementia

ENDOCRINE DISORDERS

<u>Syndrome of Inappropriate Antidiuretic Hormone Secretion (SIADH)</u>

SIADH occurs when the pituitary gland secretes high levels of antidiuretic hormone (ADH.)

Risk Factors

Risk factors include the presence of pancreatic cancer, brain tumors, leukemia, and oat cell lung carcinoma.

Signs and Symptoms

The signs and symptoms of SIADH include fluid retention, hyponatremia resulting from increased sodium excretion, hypo-osmolality (dilute plasma) and aldostereone suppression. Some of the symptoms are lethargy, mental status and mood changes in mood, and irritability.

Treatment

Non-pharmacological and pharmacological interventions aim to prevent life-threatening complications like pulmonary edema, cerebral edema, and cerebral herniation. At times, a surgical removal of a tumor is indicated; other treatments can include increased fluid intake, demeclocycline (Declomycin) to increase urinary output, lithium carbonate to decrease the effects of antidiuretic hormone, and hypertonic intravenous saline solutions.

Nurses must be aware of the warning signs of SIADH, and they must be alert to the fact that altered mental status may place the client at great risk for injury in the absence of special safety measures.

Related Nursing Diagnoses

- At risk for cerebral edema and alterations of mental status r/t decreased plasma osmolality and fluid excesses
- At risk for injury r/t SIADH

Diabetes

Diabetes mellitus, a chronic endocrine disorder that adversely affects carbohydrate, protein and fat metabolism, is the most common disease of the endocrine system and a commonly occurring comorbitity for many clients.

The different types of diabetes are:

- Type 1 diabetes mellitus, referred to as insulin-dependent diabetes in the past, is associated with some viruses, genetics, toxins, and antibodies that attack the islet of Langerhans cells. This type of diabetes is typically asymptomatic until about 90% of the pancreatic beta cells have been destroyed. Type 1 diabetes occurs most often among young people less than 30 years of age and among lean people without obesity. Clients with Type 1 diabetes are insulin dependent; absolute insulin deficiencies occur.

- Type 2 diabetes mellitus, also known as non-insulin-dependent diabetes and as adult-onset diabetes in the past, is primarily associated with obesity. This type of diabetes leads to defective insulin actions and impaired insulin secretion. More and more children are developing this disorder than in the past. Type 2 diabetes usually occurs among older populations after the age of 40, particularly when they are obese, sedentary, and have poor nutritional habits. Pathophysiologically, relative insulin deficiencies occur because the body is not able to use natural insulin effectively. These deficiencies adversely affect the liver, adipose tissue and skeletal muscle.

- Gestational diabetes mellitus occurs during pregnancy and often disappears after delivery. Other types of diabetes are associated with disorders such as pancreatic disease, endocrinopathies, some genetic syndromes, insulin receptor disorders, and the use of drugs or chemicals such as phenytoin, furosemide, epinephrine, corticosteroids, lithium, and glucagon.

Signs and Symptoms

The classic signs and symptoms associated with diabetes include polydypsia, polyphagia, polyuria, weight loss, fatigue, somnolence, and visual changes.

Treatment

The treatment of diabetes varies according to the type of diabetes and the patient's clinical status. The treatment of Type 1 includes insulin, exercise and diet. The treatment of Type II diabetes includes oral hypoglycemic drugs, diet, weight loss and exercise; insulin may become necessary when the type II diabetic client does not control their blood glucose with diet and exercise.

When diabetes is not successfully treated, a number of acute and chronic complications can occurs. Some of the acute complications include hyperglycemic hyperosmolar nonketotic coma, hypoglycemia, coma, seizures, diabetic ketoacidosis, and death. Some of the chronic complications are neuropathy, nephropathy, macrovascular complications, dyslipidemia, atherosclerosis, retinopathy, hypertension and problems with the feet such as neuropathy, numbness and infections.

Related Nursing Diagnoses

- Imbalanced nutrition: less than body requirements r/t inability of the body to use glucose (type 1); or excessive intake of nutrients (type 2)
- Risk for inefficient tissue perfusion and other long term complications r/t diabetes

II. PAIN MANAGEMENT

INTRODUCTION TO THE NURSING PROCESS

The nursing process is a form of problem solving. It is a systematic, ongoing, cyclical, dynamic, goal-directed, client-centered problem-solving approach to nursing care. It provides nurses with a systematic, logical, coherent and complete framework to address patient care needs.

The nursing process has a series of interrelated and interconnected phases that move seamlessly toward identifying and meeting the needs of clients and/or their significant others. Every phase of the nursing process affects all of the other phases of the nursing process. Data collected during one phase provides information and data that must be considered during the next phase. For example, the nurse uses data collected during the assessment phase during the analysis phase; and the evaluation phase, which is the fifth phase of the nursing process, provides data and information that is useful for the assessment phase, the first phase of the nursing process.

The five dynamic phases of the nursing process are:

1. Assessment
2. Diagnosing
3. Planning
4. Implementation
5. Evaluation

All phases of the nursing process are done with the active collaboration and participation of the client, and other people as the client chooses.

Assessment

Data that is related to the client, family members and significant others, is collected during the assessment phase of the nursing process. This data is also organized, validated with the client and others, and documented.

Diagnosis

This phase of the nursing process involves professional critical thinking in order to:

- Analyze the data and information that was collected during the assessment phase
- Identify any health related risk factors
- Determine health related concerns and problems
- Determine the strengths, as well as the weaknesses, of the client and others
- Identify and generate accurate and appropriate nursing diagnoses relating to both actual and potential health problems.

Planning

During the planning phase of nursing, the nurse determines and establishes priorities, generates the expected outcomes of care, or goals, and selects scientifically sound interventions to meet these goals.

Implementation

Implementation is the actual performance of interventions. However, during this phase, the nurse delegates some aspects of care to others, supervises the care rendered by others and reassesses client responses to the planned interventions.

Evaluation

The evaluation phase, closely similar to the assessment phase, cyclically returns data and information into the assessment phase of the nursing process. Evaluation data, which reflect the client's current condition, is compared and contrasted to the preestablished expected outcomes of care, which were established during the planning phase of the nursing process. The nurse then makes a determination about goal achievement. Were the goals completely met? Were the goals only partially met? Were the goals not met at all? After these determinations, the nurse decides to continue, modify, or discontinue part of the plan of care.

A COMPREHENSIVE PAIN ASSESSMENT

Assessment data can be primary or secondary data. Primary data is provided by the client themselves; secondary data is collected from other sources, such as previous medical records, laboratory test results and radiographic studies. Data can also be classified as subjective and objective. Subjective data is not measurable or observable and it typically consists of the client's own words. For example, a statement from the client about their pain is an example of subjective data. Objective data, on the other hand, is measurable and empirically observable. Vital signs, for example, are objective data.

Pain can be acute or chronic; pain has emotional and sensory components. Sympathetic nervous system effects accompany acute pain, such as increased respiratory and pulse rates and diaphoresis, as well as emotional effects like anxiety. Emotional depression and changes such as anorexia and fatigue accompany chronic pain.

Some of the questions to ask a client to assess their pain include:

- How would you describe your symptoms?
- When did the symptoms begin?
- What precipitates it?
- What relieves it?
- What makes it worse?
- How often does the pain occur?
- Where is the pain?
- What is the character (crushing, sore, etc.), intensity (on a pain scale from 1 to 10), the quality (color of the sputum, etc.) and the quantity (amount of drainage, etc.) of the presenting symptom or concern?

Pain can be localized or diffuse. Pain can be referred, and can also be described as visceral. Referred pain originates from one part of the body but it manifests itself in another part of the body. For example, cardiac ischemic pain may not be localized in the chest or sterna area, but instead referred to the arm, shoulder and/or jaw with or without accompanying chest pain. Visceral pain is organ pain.

Pain is also characterized in terms of its duration. Acute pain has a rapid onset and brief duration. Chronic pain, on the other hand, has a prolonged duration that persists for or reoccurs for months or even years. Cancer pain, also referred to as malignant pain, and nonmalignant pain, unrelated to cancer, are different. Cancer pain can occur as the direct effects of the cancer as well as the result of a cancer treatment.

Pain can be mild, moderate or severe. Using a numeric pain rating scale from 0 to 10 with 10 being the most intensely severe pain and 0 being the absence of pain is helpful for assessing the degree of pain that the client is experiencing. A rating of 1 to 3 is usually mild pain; a rating of 4 to 6 is considered moderate pain; and a rating of more than 6 is considered severe pain.

Some pediatric and neonatal pain assessment scales, used before the child can adequately verbalize their intensity of pain include the Pre-Verbal, Early Verbal Pediatric Pain Scale (PEPPS), the Children's Hospital of Eastern Ontario Pain Scale (CHEOPS), Faces Legs Activity Cry Consolability Pain Scale (FLACC), Toddler Preschooler Postoperative Pain Scale (TPPPS), the observer Visual Analog Scale (VASobs) the Observation Scale of Behavioral Distress (OSBD), the FACES Pain Scale, the neonatal CRIES Pain Scale, the Neonatal Infant Pain Scale (NIPS) and the COMFORT Pain Scale.

Observational behavioral scales are used for children less than three years of age; self-reports of pain are used for pain assessments of children three years of age and older unless they are affected with a disorder, like a developmental disorder, or the inability to communicate their level of pain.

The Etiology of Pain

The etiology of pain is classified as physiological pain and neuropathic pain. Subcategories of physiological pain are visceral and somatic pain. Subcategories of neuropathic pain are central neuropathic, peripheral neuropathic and sympathetically mediated pain. Neuropathic pain is associated with tingling, burning, and aching. It is often chronic and perhaps the most difficult and challenging to treat.

Pain is also classified as acute and chronic. Acute pain occurs with peripheral pain receptor (A delta and C sensory nerve) activation and typically occurs with tissue injury. Chronic pain occurs with ongoing peripheral pain receptor activation and continuous tissue damage.

Types of Pain

Visceral pain is not as apparent and not as easily located as somatic pain is. Visceral pain originates from organ and surrounding tissue damage. Visceral pain can be described as cramping, aching, throbbing and pressing; visceral pain is often accompanied with client complaints such as "feeling sick." Somatic pain, on the other hand, has its etiology in the bones, skin, muscles and connective tissue. It is often described as being sharp.

Neuropathic pain results from neurological damage or disease. Central neuropathic pain occurs as the result of damage to the central nervous system, as occurs with spinal cord injuries. Peripheral neuropathic pain arises from the peripheral nervous system, as occurs with neuropathy, carpal tunnel syndrome and phantom pain after an amputation. This pain is described as stabbing and burning. Lastly, sympathetically mediated pain has its etiology in a pathological connection between the sympathetic nervous system and nerve pain fibers.

Factors that Influence the Experience of Pain

Many factors affect pain, the fifth vital sign, and the pain experience including ethnicity, culture, developmental stage along the lifespan, the presence or absence of supports that the client has, past pain experiences, and the person's individual and personal definitions of pain.

Intractable pain is quite severe and not readily amenable to treatment. Fear and depression also affect the client's experience of pain and they can also result as a complication, or consequence, of pain.

Related Nursing Diagnoses

- Alteration of comfort level r/t pain
- Alteration of comfort level r/t chemotherapy or radiation therapy
- At risk for depression r/t chronic pain

PHARMACOLOGICAL INTERVENTIONS

Pain Medications

Below are some of the most commonly used pain medications in pharmacological interventions.

Opioid Analgesics

Drug	Dosage	Delivery	Indicated For
Codeine	30 mg q 4-6h	Oral	Mild to moderate pain
Fentanyl	50 mcg/hour (q 72h)	Oral, nasal, transdermal	Breakthrough pain
Hydrocodone	5-10 mg q 4-6h	Oral	Hydrocodone is available only in combination with other ingredients. Some hydrocodone products are used to relieve moderate to severe pain; other hydrocodone products are used to relieve cough.
Hydromorphone	2 mg 4-6h	Oral, injection, and rectal	Moderate to severe pain.
Methadone	2.5-5 mg BID-TID	Oral	Moderate to severe pain not relieved by non-narcotic pain relievers

Morphine	Immediate release 10 mg q 4h; sustained release 15 mg q 12h	Oral, rectal and injection	Moderate to severe pain
Oxycodone	Immediate release 5 mg q 4-6h Sustained release 10 mg q 12h	Oral	Moderate to severe pain
Oxymorphone	Immediate release 5-10 mg q 4-6h Sustained release 10 mg q 12h	Oral	Moderate to severe pain

Titrating Medications Using Baseline and Breakthrough Doses

Although the dosage of an analgesic is initially based on a number of factors, including the severity of the pain, the age of the client and the general state of health, the initial dose is often modified, or titrated, over time until increasing incremental dosages produce the desired analgesic effect without adverse side effects.

Often, during long-term treatment, the dosage can remain the same for a period of time after initial titration, with only some increases or decreases as based on the desired outcome and the presence of any adverse effects. Dosages are typically increased from 30% to 100% without fears of tolerance, when the pain is not relieved with the current dosage.

Breakthrough doses, also referred to as rescue dosages, are what are known as *pro re nata* (prn) doses. The Latin means, "As circumstances arise." Prn doses are for breakthrough pain and sporadic increases in the client's level of pain. For example, an additional dose of morphine that is typically 10% of the total daily dosage of morphine may be given to the client when pain has broken though shortly before the next scheduled dosage of morphine is given.

Breakthrough, or rescue dosages, are indicated when pain occurs as the result of an incident like out of bed activity, when the pain is spontaneous without a known incident, and when the pain occurs shortly before the next scheduled dose. Breakthrough doses are typically ordered prn every hour. For example, a rescue dosage for a client who takes 10 mg of morphine q 4 h with a total daily dosage of 60 mg would have a rescue, or breakthrough, dosage of 6 mg (10% of 60 mg) of morphine every 1 h prn (as needed.)

Administering Analgesic Medications

The "Ten Rights of Medication Administration" are *the right, or correct*:

1. Medication
2. Dosage
3. Time
4. Route
5. Client
6. Client education
7. Documentation
8. Right to refuse
9. Assessment
10. Evaluation

Some groups of patients are more at risk for medication errors. Some client populations that are at greatest risk are infants, children and the elderly, as well as members of a population that have a language barrier, cognitive impairment, decreased level of consciousness, sensory disorder and/or developmental or psychiatric disorder.

Accurate identification is necessary during all aspects of nursing care, especially during medication administration. At least two (2) unique identifiers, other than room number, must be used. Some examples of unique identifiers include a unique code number, the person's first, middle and last name and/or complete date of birth including year, an encoded bar code with at least 2 unique identifiers imbedded into it and a photograph.

DOSAGE EQUIVALENTS

Measurement Systems

The three systems of measurement used in pharmacology are the household measurement system, the metric system and the apothecary system.

The household measurement system is more often utilized in the outpatient setting, like a local pharmacy, rather than within medical settings. It is the least precise and exact of all the measurement systems. It includes measurements for drops, teaspoons, tablespoons, ounces, cups, pints, quart, gallons, and pounds.

The apothecary system of measurement is the oldest forms of measurement; it is rarely used today. The weight units of measurement in this system include grain (gr), scruple, dram, ounce and pound. The volume units of measurement are the minim (m), fluid dram, a fluid ounce, a pint, a quart and a gallon.

The metric system is the most commonly used measurement system in pharmacology. The volume measurements for this system include liters (L), cubic milliliters (ml) and cubic centimeter (cc.) The units of weight in this system include kilograms (kg), grams (g), milligrams (mg) and micrograms (mcg.)

Each system can be converted to another system when the proper equivalents are used for this mathematical calculation. The ten most commonly used equivalents are:

- 1 Kg = 1,000 g
- 1 Kg = 2.2 lbs
- 1 L = 1,000 mL
- 1 g = 1,000 mg
- 1 mg = 1,000 mcg
- 1 gr = 60 mg
- 1 oz. = 30 g or 30 mL
- 1 tsp = 5 mL
- 1 lb = 454 g
- 1 tbsp = 15 mL

Example of an Oral Dosage Calculation

Doctor's order: 500 mg of medication once a day
Medication label: 1 tablet = 125 mg

How many tablets should be administered daily?

In this problem, you have to determine how many tablets the patient will take if the doctor's order is for 500 mg a day and the tablets are manufactured in 125 mg each.

This problem can be set up and calculated as shown below.

500 mg: x tablets = 125 mg: 1 tablet

Or as:

$$\frac{500 mg}{x} = \frac{125 mg}{1 \text{ tablet}}$$

Then you multiply: 500 mg x 1 = 500 mg

125 x = 500 mg

$$X = \frac{500}{125}$$

OR

500 ÷ 125 = 4 tablets

Examples of Intramuscular and Subcutaneous Dosage Calculations

Intramuscular:

Doctor's order: 10 mg/kg IM tid
Patient's weight: 230 lbs
Medication label: 250 mg/1 mL

How many milliliters need to be administered?

$$\frac{230 \text{ lbs}}{X kg} = \frac{2.2 \text{ lbs}}{1 \text{ kg}}$$

2.2 X = 230

$$X = \frac{230}{2.2}$$

230 ÷ 2.2 = 104.54 kg

The patient's weight can be rounded off to: 105 kg because the tenths place (5) is equal to or more than 5.

The next step is to figure out how many milliliters the patient will get in each of the three doses per day.

$$\frac{10 \text{ mg}}{1 \text{ kg}} = \frac{X \text{ mg}}{105 \text{ kg}}$$

1 X = 105 × 10

105 × 10 = 1050 mg

In the final step, you will need to calculate how many milliliters you need to administer the ordered number of milligrams.

$$\frac{250 \text{ mg}}{1 \text{ mL}} = \frac{1050 \text{ mg}}{X \text{ mL}}$$

250 X = 1050 = $\frac{1050}{250}$

1050 ÷ 250 = 4.2 mL

Answer: 4.2 mL

Subcutaneous

Doctor's order: 2,500 units subcutaneously
Medication label: 5,000 units/mL

How many milliliters will you administer to this patient?

$$\frac{X \text{ mL}}{2,500 \text{ Units}} = \frac{1 \text{ mL}}{5,000 \text{ Units}}$$

5,000 X = 2,500

X = $\frac{2,500}{5,000}$

2,500 ÷ 5,000 = 0.5

Answer: 0.5 mL

Example of Intravenous Fluid Rate Calculation

Doctor's order: 0.9% Na Cl solution at 50 mL per hour
How many gtts per minute should you administer if the tube delivers 20 gtts/mL?

X gtts per min = $\frac{50 \times 20}{60} = \frac{1000}{60}$ = 16.6 gtts

Rounded off to: 17 gtts/min

ADMINISTERING ADJUVANT MEDICATIONS

Adjuvant medications have a potentiating effect when given with analgesic medications. The nonsteroidal anti-inflammatory drugs (NSAIDs), corticosteroids, anticonvulsant medications and antidepressants are the most commonly used adjuvant medications.

According to the World Health Organization (WHO), pain should be treated in a stepwise manner. The WHO has developed a Pain Ladder to describe these steps. The first step includes nonopioid medications, followed by mild opioids, like codeine, and then strong opioids like morphine. Adjuvant medications help decrease the pain and they also are useful for decreasing anxiety associated with the pain or another cause.

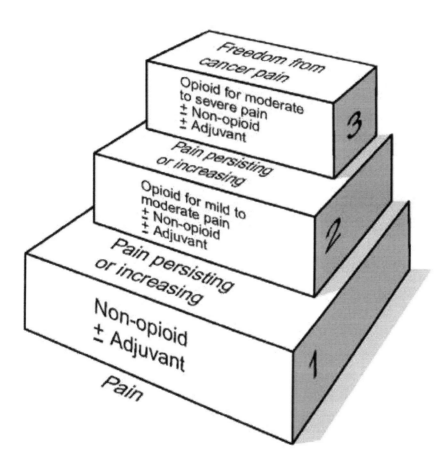

Non-steroidal Anti-Inflammatory Drugs (NSAIDS)

Drug	Dosage Range	Delivery	Indicated For:
Naproxen	250-500 mg q 12h	Oral, rectal	Pain related to inflammatory conditions and chronic inflammatory conditions
Naproxen Na	275-550 mg q 12h	Oral	Pain and inflammation from muscular injuries
Oxaprozin	600-1200 mg q 24 h	Oral	Pain, stiffness and inflammation associated with rheumatoid and osteoarthritis
Aspirin	650-1000 mg q 4-6h	Oral	Pain, fever, and inflammation
Diflunisal	250-500 mg q 8-12h	Oral	Mild to moderate pain and inflammation
Salsalate	750-2000 mg q 12h	Oral	Pain, tenderness, swelling, and stiffness
Meclofenamate	50-100 mg q 6-8h	Oral	Mild to moderate pain, tenderness, swelling, and stiffness

Mefenamic acid	250 mg q 6h	Oral	Mild to moderate pain relief
Ketorolac (Toradol)	15-30 mg IV or IM q 6h or 20 followed by 10 mg q 4-6h	Oral, IM, IV and IV	Short-term management (up to 5 days) of moderately severe acute pain that otherwise would require narcotics
Diclofenac	50-100 mg, followed by 50 mg q 8h	Oral	Mild to moderate pain, fever and inflammation
Etodolac	200-400 mg q 6-8h	Oral	Inflammation and pain relief
Indomethacin	25-50 mg q 6-8h	Oral and rectal	Fever, pain and inflammation
Sulindac	150-200 mg q 12h	Oral	Used for treating pain, fever, and inflammation.

Piroxicam	20-40 mg q 24h	Oral	Fever, pain, and inflammation
Acetaminophen	650-1000 mg q 6-8h	Oral	Acetaminophen relieves pain by elevating the pain threshold and it is also an antipyretic
Fenoprofen	200-600 mg q 6h	Oral	Mild to moderate pain, tenderness, swelling, and stiffness
Flurbiprofen	50-200 mg q 12h	Oral	Pain, tenderness, swelling, and stiffness relief
Ibuprofen	400mg q 4h to 800 mg q6h	Oral	Prescription strength and over-the-counter preparations are available. It relieves pain, tenderness, swelling, stiffness and fever

Ketoprofen	25-50 mg q 6-8h	Oral	Prescription strength and over-the-counter preparations are available.
			It is used to relieve pain, tenderness, swelling, stiffness, minor aches and pains from headaches, menstrual periods, toothaches, and backaches as well as an antipyretic
Celecoxib	100-200 mg q 12h	Oral	Pain, tenderness, swelling and stiffness

Anticonvulsants

Drug Name	Dosage Range and Route	Indicated For:
Carbamazepine	Oral dose two to four times a day Extended release tablet twice a day	Chronic low back pain, cancer pain, and restless leg syndrome
Gabapentin	Oral once every 12 hours Extended release once a day	Chronic low back pain, cancer pain, and restless leg syndrome
Phenytoin	Oral two or three times a day Extended release capsules 1 to 3 times a day	Chronic low back pain, and cancer pain
Pregabalin	Oral capsule once daily	Chronic low back pain, cancer pain, and neuropathic pain
Topiramate	Oral twice a day (same time each day preferably morning and evening)	Chronic low back pain, cancer pain and prevention of migraine headaches

Carbamazepine	Oral two to four times a day and extended release tablet twice a day, and extended-release capsule twice a day	Cancer pain and facial nerve pain
Levetiracetam	Oral twice a day at the same time each day preferably in the morning and evening	Cancer pain
Oxcarbazepine	Oral twice a day at the same time each day preferably in the morning and evening	Cancer pain
Zonisamide	Oral capsule once or twice a day at the same time each day	Cancer pain
Valproic acid	Oral once a day	Restless leg syndrome

Corticosteroids

Drug	Dosage Range and Route	Indicated For:
Prednisone	One to four times a day or once every other day	Used alone or with other medications to treat certain types of cancer, arthritis, severe allergic reactions, multiple sclerosis, lupus, other conditions
Methylprednisolone	Oral and sodium succinate injection	Inflammation relief and treatment of certain forms of cancer, arthritis; skin, blood, kidney, eye, thyroid, and intestinal disorders, severe allergies, and asthma
Fluticasone and salmeterol	Oral twice daily and nasal inhalation once or twice daily	Oral inhalation is used to prevent asthmatic, chest tightness, wheezing, coughing, and dyspnea Nasal spray used to treat the symptoms of seasonal and perennial allergic rhinitis and perennial non-allergic rhinitis.

Beclomethasone	Oral inhalation three to four times daily and nasal inhalation two to four times daily	Prevention of wheezing, shortness of breath, coughing, and chest tightness caused by severe asthma and other lung diseases.
Hydrocortisone	Oral, topical and injection	Inflammation relief and treatment of kidney, eye, thyroid, and intestinal disorders (e.g., colitis); severe allergies; and asthma; also treats certain types of cancer.
Budesonide and formoterol	Oral capsule in the morning, nasal sprays once or twice daily and oral inhalation powder once or twice a day.	Oral is used to treat Crohn's disease Nasal spray is used to treat symptoms of stuffiness and runny nose due to allergies and the prevention of wheezing, shortness of breath, and dyspnea caused by severe asthma and other lung diseases

Mometasone	Oral inhalation powder once or twice daily; nasal inhalation spray one spray in each nostril one time a day; and topical once a day.	The inhalation form prevents dyspnea, chest tightness, wheezing, and coughing caused by asthma Nasal inhalation treats and prevents the nasal symptoms of seasonal and perennial allergies, including runny nose, sneezing, and itchy nose Topical relieves the itching and inflammation of numerous skin conditions
Triamcinolone	Oral, and nasal spray once daily	Oral form is used to treat certain types of cancer, inflammation, and the treatment of certain forms of arthritis, skin, blood, kidney, eye, thyroid, and intestinal disorders (e.g., colitis) as well as severe allergies and asthma Triamcinolone nasal spray is used to treat the symptoms of seasonal, and perennial allergic rhinitis and perennial non-allergic rhinitis

Tricyclic Antidepressants

Drug	Dosage Range and Route	Indicated For:
Amitriptyline	Oral one to four times a day	Neck pain, low back pain, chronic pelvic pain and chronic pain syndrome
Doxepin	Topical and oral capsule one to three times a day	Neck pain, low back pain, chronic pelvic pain, and chronic pain syndrome
Imipramine	Oral	Neck pain, low back pain, chronic pelvic pain, and chronic pain syndrome
Desipramine	Oral	Low back pain, and chronic pain syndrome
Nortriptyline	Oral	Low back pain, and chronic pain syndrome

| Maprotiline | Oral | Low back pain |
| Trazodone | Oral | Chronic pelvic pain |

INTERACTIONS AND SIDE EFFECTS

Basic Pharmacological Definitions of Terms

Therapeutic or desired effect: A therapeutic effect is the primary, expected effect of a specific medication. For example, the therapeutic effect of metoprolol is to lower blood pressure.

Side effects: A side effect of a medication is a secondary, not primary, effect of a medication. Some side effects are desirable, others are minor, and some can be major.

Idiosyncratic effects: Unexpected side effects that are peculiar and specific to a particular client. When a sedative makes a person agitated, rather than sedated, this is an idiosyncratic effect.

Cumulative effects: The buildup of the medication in the client's system because of impaired excretion or metabolism of the drug, which can lead to toxic effects.

Adverse effects: The most serious side effects of drugs that lead to the immediate discontinuation of the medication. Adverse effects must be reported.

Drug toxicity: An over dosage of a medication that occurs when the client's metabolism and/or excretion is impaired.

Potentiating effect: A synergistic effect results from the combination of two or more drugs where the effects of one, or both, are increased.

Inhibiting effect: An inhibiting effect is one that results from the combination of two or more drugs where the effects of one or both, are decreased.

Drug allergy: An antigen-antibody immunologic response to a medication. All clients must be assessed for any drug sensitivities or allergies.

Anaphylactic reaction: This is the most severe of all medication allergy responses, which can be life threatening. The throat and tongue swell, obstructing the airway.

Drug tolerance: This often occurs when a client has been receiving an opioid for an extended period. The client needs increasing doses of the drug in order to achieve the therapeutic effect.

Drug interaction: Drugs can interact with a number of things including other prescribed drugs, over-the-counter drug, foods, herbs, and other natural substances.

All medications have intended uses, or indications, for use; and some medications are contraindicated for certain patients. For example, a medication can be contraindicated for clients who have an allergy to the medication, hepatic disease and/or renal disease as well as lactating and pregnant women. Other medications may, at certain times, be allowed with caution; for instance, a medication may be used with caution among the elderly.

Medications can interact with a number of substances. Some interactions include those with other medications including "over-the-counter" drugs, foods, and lifestyle choices, such as alcohol use, supplements and other natural substances. Virtually all medications have side effects. Nausea and vomiting are the most common side effects; most side effects are simply troublesome but others, referred to as adverse effects, can be life threatening. There are still more medications associated with toxic effects. For example, tinnitus is a sign of toxicity associated with aspirin and bradycardia is associated with digitalis toxicity. Lastly, clients can experience adverse effects from medications. These adverse effects are often very serious and sometimes life threatening. Nurses must monitor clients for their responses to medications and the presence of any side effects or adverse reactions.

NON-PHARMACOLOGICAL INTERVENTIONS

Responding to Psychosocial, Cultural and Spiritual Issues Related to Pain

A number of client-related factors affect the experience pain, including psychosocial, cultural, and spiritual issues. Some cultures and ethnic groups are highly accepting of pain and expression of pain among members of both genders, others may have cultural norms that shun male expressions while accepting female expressions of pain, and still others that may be characterized by stoicism and denials of pain.

Spiritual beliefs also affect pain and expressions of pain. Some religious beliefs lead followers to view pain as a way to make amends for our failings and shortcomings, and others may view pain or illness as punishment for sins and wrongdoings.

Some of the psychosocial factors that affect pain include level of development, the support of others, past pain experiences, fear, anxiety, and the person's personal perceptions of pain.

Nurses should attempt to modify these factors so they facilitate, rather than add to, the pain that the client is experiencing. For example, fear and anxiety can be alleviated with knowledge about the origins of the pain and with relaxation techniques, for example. All cultures, ethnic and religious groups should be assessed in terms of their pain-related norms and practices in order to encourage the expressions of pain and the acceptance of pain interventions.

Implementing and Facilitating Non-Pharmacological Interventions

The number and variety of nonpharmacological interventions including complementary, alternative and integrative modalities are numerous and varied. Some clients prefer some methods and modalities over others but there are so many options that at least one or more may be highly beneficial for the client and significant others. For example, massage and relaxation techniques can relieve pain and anxiety.

Magnets

Although the benefits of magnets for pain are not scientifically substantiated, according to the National Institutes of Health (NIH), they can be associated with some undesired side effects. However, some people claim that they benefit from them. Some clients report relief of back pain, foot pain, arthritis pain and the pain associated with fibromyalgia.

Magnets, typically made of a metal like iron and alloys or mixtures of metals and/or non-metals, produce a magnetic field of different strengths as measured in terms of gauss. Magnets for pain relief typically have a strength of 300 to 5,000 gauss. To put this strength into context, these magnets are stronger than the magnetic field of the Earth and less than the magnets used for an MRI.

Magnets may not be safe among clients with an insulin pump or pacemaker; and they should not be used in lieu of more traditional and conventional pain relief measures.

Chiropractic Services

Many Americans seek chiropractic services, particularly when they are affected with acute or chronic back pain, headaches, and/or neck pain. Chiropractors use spinal manipulation and other treatments, including deep massage, to support the proper alignment of the body. It is believed that this manipulation restores mobility and decreases pain.

Chiropractic care is usually considered safe, but clients who have spinal cord compressions or who are taking anticoagulants should not use chiropractic spinal manipulation.

Homeopathy

Like other alternative treatments, homeopathic approaches to pain are not substantiated in the literature and, despite the fact that homeopathic remedies are regulated by the U.S. Food and Drug Administration, this regulatory agency does not confirm their safety and effectiveness. Some of these remedies can also have adverse side effects.

Practitioners of homeopathic medicine believe that disorders and diseases can be treated with lower, highly diluted dosages rather than higher doses of a substance such as a plant, mineral or animal source. Some substances include low doses of mountain herb, red onions, white arsenic, stinging nettle and belladonna.

Massage

Massage decreases stress and pain. Relaxation techniques, soothing music and soft lighting, combined with massage, is a great way to help to alleviate stress and pain to promote sleep, rest and circulation. It also conveys caring and compassion as part of the nurse-client relationship and gives the nurse a chance to speak with the client about their concerns. Massage can include hand massage, back massage, foot soaking and massage, and neck massage. A warm lotion or oil is used for massage.

Meditation

Meditation is thought to reduce fatigue, stress and anxiety. During meditation, the client should be instructed to concentrate on one's breathing while repeating positive and calming phrases in one's mind. Meditation is spiritual, whereas prayer is often religious – however, many Christians, including Catholics, Baptists and numerous evangelical denominations may react negatively to the suggestion of meditation, so it is important to be sensitive to the client's beliefs.

Prayer

Prayers can be formal or informal as well as religious and non-religious in nature.

Heat and Cold Applications

Heat and cold applications can be quite helpful in the reduction of pain. Heat can be helpful in reducing the pain associated with sore muscles. It can be applied with a heating pad, gel packet, warm water bottle or a hot bath or shower. Heat should not be used for more than ten minutes at a time.

Cold can help relive or ease the pain in a patient by numbing it for a period. Cold can be administered with cold gel packs, frozen peas or ice cubes wrapped in a cloth. This, like the heat, should be used for a maximum of ten minutes.

Deep Breathing

Deep breathing techniques are shown to be effective with tension, pain, anxiety and fatigue.

Progressive Muscular Relaxation

Progressive muscular relaxation (PMR) therapy aims to reduce tension, to lower perceived stress, to decrease pain and to induce relaxation in the patient. It involves progressively tensing and releasing major skeletal muscle groups. Its goal is to reduce the stimulation of the autonomic and central nervous system and to increase parasympathetic activity.

It has been reported that patients who use progressive muscular relaxation experience a reduction in their state of anxiety, pain, symptoms of depression, and improve their sleeping habits as well as their overall quality of life.

Distraction

According to the American Cancer Society, distraction means turning your attention to something other than the pain. Distraction aims to manage mild pain and pain that occurs before an ordered analgesic medication takes effect. Some forms of distraction are watching television, talking on the telephone, or other things that can help the patient take their minds off the pain they are experiencing.

Imagery

Imagery, also referred to as guided imagery or visualization, is a set of mental exercises designed to allow the mind to influence the health and wellbeing of the body. The patient creates a kind of purposeful daydream by imagining sights, smells, tastes or other sensations. Imagery is helpful in reducing stress, anxiety, depression, pain, and hypertension.

Biofeedback

Biofeedback is a method of treatment in which the patient is able to use monitoring devices to help consciously control physical processes that are normally controlled automatically. For example, temperature, heart rate, sweating, blood pressure, muscle tension and sweating can be controlled.

It has been shown that biofeedback can help patients with chronic pain, sleep difficulties and it can help to improve the patient's overall quality of life.

Hypnosis

Self-hypnosis and hypnosis produce a state that includes relaxation and deep concentration. It is helpful for reducing pain, fear, anxiety and fatigue among oncology clients.

Transcutaneous Nerve Stimulation (TENS)

A transcutaneous nerve stimulator, also referred to as a TENS unit, is used as a method of pain relief. TENS transmits low-voltage electrical impulses through electrodes placed on the skin on or around where the pain is. This nerve stimulation activates the body's pain modulatory pathways, thus decreasing the pain.

Acupuncture

This ancient Chinese medical treatment uses very thin needles, which are placed into the skin, and it can help to reduce pain, nausea and vomiting.

Acupressure

Acupressure is similar to acupuncture, but it uses pressure instead of needless. It can be quite helpful in the treatment of anticipatory nausea.

Reiki

Reiki is another complementary healing approach. The therapist places their hands above the person, or lightly on the person, to facilitate the client's own healing processes and responses. This Eastern therapy is based on the belief that energy supports healing. A limited number of studies have been done relating to Reiki and its benefits; some of these studies indicate that there may be some benefits in terms of the symptoms of cancer, depression, pain, fibromyalgia, and depression.

Music Therapy

Music Therapy intends to enhance the client's emotional, physical, cognitive and overall sense of wellbeing. Music therapists engage clients with singing, movement to music, creating music and listening to music. Many clients, particularly those who cannot speak, enjoy music as a form of alternative communication and stress reduction.

The four general types of music therapy are receptive, improvisation, recreative and creative. Receptive therapy includes things like listening to music and moving in rhythm or dancing; improvisation includes the active creation of music using voice sounds and musical instruments; recreative musical therapy includes recreational social activities like singing in a chorus; compositional music therapy includes creative song writing and musical compositions.

Mind-Body Exercises

Mind-body exercises combine deep focused breathing, movement and meditation. These exercises can help the oncology client combat stress, depression and fatigue. Yoga and tai chi are two examples of mind-body exercises.

Herbs

Herbs and dietary supplements are helpful for many oncology patients. Some herbs reduce vomiting and nausea, others help to decrease pain and fatigue. For example, astragalus, which comes from the astragalus plant's root, can boost the immune system. Vitamins A, C, E and coenzyme Q 10 may provide some protection against cancer.

Many herbs and supplements are not documented in the literature as being scientifically effective against pain, and some can have possible side effects. It is therefore necessary to instruct your clients about the need to consult with their physician prior to the use of these substances.

Evaluation

All clients are evaluated for the side effects, interactions, efficacy and complications relating to all pharmacological and non-pharmacological interventions for pain. For example, the level of pain should be assessed prior to the administration of a pain drug and the level of pain must also be assessed after the medication was administered in order to determine whether or not it was effective in treating the pain.

Similarly, clients should be evaluated for the presence of any side effects or adverse reactions and/or interactions with other medications (potentiating or inhibiting), foods, and alternative treatments such as herbs and vitamins.

III. SYMPTOM MANAGEMENT

NEUROLOGICAL SYMPTOMS

Aphasia

There are two major types of aphasia: receptive aphasia, also referred to as Wernicke's aphasia, and expressive aphasia, which is often referred to as Broca's aphasia. Receptive aphasia impairs the person's ability to recognize and comprehend words, language and forms of written communication. Expressive aphasia impairs the ability of the person to express and create words and writings despite the fact that they can comprehend words.

Signs and Symptoms

The signs and symptoms of aphasia vary according to the specific type of aphasia and its severity. Some of these signs and symptoms include slow speech, often spoken in short phrases, fluent speech that is jumbled and not logical, impaired writing and repetition skills, altered auditory comprehension, problems with reading, and an inability to repeat words and phrases.

Aphasia is often diagnosed after other possible causes, such as delirium, hearing, visual and motor writing abilities, are ruled out. Formal assessments can be done with a speech and language therapist using the Western Aphasia, Boston Diagnostic Aphasia, and Naming tests, among others.

Treatment

Speech and language therapists and augmentative communication devices, like pictures and communication boards, are often helpful.

Possible Nursing Diagnoses

- Impaired comprehension relating to receptive aphasia
- Impaired speech and writing skills relating to expressive aphasia
- Potential for grieving secondary to the loss of ability to communicate with others as a result of aphasia
- Anxiety related to a situational crisis secondary to aphasia

Dysphagia

Dysphagia is difficulty swallowing or expending an excessive amount of time and effort to move food and/or liquid from the mouth to the stomach. In some severe cases, the client may not be able to swallow at all and if the problem is persistent it can be indicative of a serious medical condition that requires treatment. Dysphagia can affect people of any age, but it is more commonly seen in the elderly.

Signs and Symptoms

There are a variety of signs and symptoms that can be associated with dysphagia, which include not being able to swallow, odynophagia or pain while swallowing, drooling, frequent heartburn, coughing or gagging when swallowing, the sensation of food getting stuck in one's throat, chest, or behind one's breastbone, hoarseness, regurgitation, and unexpected weight loss. If breathing is ever obstructed, emergency help is necessary.

Treatment

The treatment for dysphagia depends on the cause. If the client has oropharyngeal dysphagia they are most commonly treated by a speech or swallowing therapist who can assist the client with exercises and swallowing techniques.

Clients with esophageal dysphagia can be treated with esophageal dilation, surgery, and medications. Severe cases of dysphagia, which affect the client's ability to safely eat and/or drink the adequate amount necessary, may require specialized liquid diets or even feeding tubes.

Related Nursing Diagnoses

- At risk for aspiration r/t dysphagia
- Imbalanced nutrition r/t dysphagia

Levels of Consciousness

Levels of consciousness can change as the result of several causes some of which are structural and some of which are classified as metabolic. Examples of structural or biological causes of decreased levels of consciousness include infections, cancer, including brain tumors, intracerebral hemorrhage, vascular insults like a cerebrovascular accident, and trauma like a closed head injury. Some metabolic causes of decreased levels of consciousness include seizures, hypoxic encephalopathies, as caused by heart failure and hypertension, systemic metabolic problems like hypoglycemia, ketoacidosis, toxins, and changes in body temperature with extremes of hyperthermia and hypothermia.

Signs and Symptoms

The six levels of consciousness are alert, confused, lethargic, obtunded, stuporous and comatose. Alert clients follow commands and answer questions appropriateness with minimal stimulation. Confused clients are not oriented to their environment, and they may lack good judgment and they need cues in order to respond to commands. Lethargic clients are drowsy but verbal or tactile stimulation can rouse them. Obtunded patients respond slowly and only with repeated stimulation, and stuporous clients minimally respond to vigorous stimulation and they may not verbally respond to this stimuli with anything more than a moan. Lastly, comatose clients are completely unresponsive to external stimuli.

The three states associated with altered levels of consciousness are a persistent vegetative state, locked-in syndrome and brain death. A client in a persistent vegetative state demonstrates no cognitive functioning beyond basic functions like a sleep-wake cycle and eye opening. Clients with locked-in syndrome retain cognitive functioning but are unable to function beyond communicating with eye movements; they are typically aware of their surroundings. Brain death is achieved when there is a known cause of the coma, the coma is irreversible, complete unresponsiveness to eternal stimuli, a complete loss of all brainstem reflexes, and the absence of all respiratory function.

The Glasgow Coma Scales for adults and children are standardized assessment tools for altered levels of consciousness. These scales assess motor responses, verbal responses and eye opening. The Rancho Los Amigos scale is used to determine a client's cognitive level of functioning. This scale ranges from I to VIII, with I as the total lack of all responsiveness to all stimulation and VIII as alert, oriented, appropriate and purposeful.

Treatment

Treatment includes the correction of the underlying cause, when possible. For example, hypoglycemia can be treated and reversed. When correction of an underlying disorder is not possible, supportive medical and nursing care are indicated.

Possible Nursing Diagnoses

- Ineffective breathing r/t decreased level of consciousness
- Disturbed thought processes r/t decreased level of consciousness
- At risk for injury r/t decreased level of consciousness

Myoclonus

Myoclonus, also known as myoclonus dystonia, typically appears in childhood and adolescence, and is sometimes triggered by caffeine, sudden noise or stress. It appears to be genetic in origin for many, but for others, it can be a symptom of a cerebellar disorder like Alzheimer's disease (cortical myoclonus.) Those with myoclonus are at risk for anxiety, panic attacks and depression.

Signs and Symptoms

The signs and symptoms include quick, nonrhythmic, involuntary muscle jerking of the upper body, trunk, neck, legs, and hand muscles.

Treatment

Levetiracetam appears to be effective with cortical myoclonus, whereas clonazepam remains the only first-line therapeutic option in subcortical and spinal myoclonus.

Possible Nursing Diagnoses

- At risk for injury r/t myoclonus
- Poor self esteem r/t myoclonus

Neuropathies and Paresthesia

Neuropathy consists of nerve ischemia, or death, as the result of a combination of metabolic changes within the cells that alter nerve fiber functioning. It is common among diabetic clients and the direct effect of high glucose levels on nerve neurons and ischemia in the microvascular circulation.

There are multiple types of diabetic neuropathy, including the following:

- Symmetric polyneuropathy, which is the most commonly occurring form of diabetic neuropathy, is often referred to as the "stocking glove" type of neuropathy because it affects the hands and the feet.

- Autonomic neuropathy, which can affect all aspects of the autonomic nervous system

- Radiculopathy is classified according to the location of origin. Diabetic amyotrophy occurs when L2 through L4 (spinal lumbar nerve roots) are affected, and thoracic polyradiculopathy occurs when T4 to T12 (spinal thoracic) nerve roots are affected.

- Cranial neuropathy can adversely affect the 3rd cranial nerve (the oculomotor nerve), the 4th cranial nerve (the trochlear nerve), and the 6th cranial nerve (the abducens nerve.)

Signs and Symptoms

- Symmetric Polyneuropathy confers paresthesia, which is a feeling of tingling or pricking resulting from pressure or damage to a client's peripheral nerves, as well as dysesthesias, which is a painful or uncomfortable sense of touch, and sensory losses to touch, temperature and vibration can occur.

  These sensory deficits can lead to foot ulcerations, infections, which are difficult to treat because of the diabetes, fractures, subluxation, which is a partial or complete dislocation of a bone at the joint, and the destruction of the normal foot anatomy, which is referred to as Charcot joint.

Small fiber neuropathy is marked with the preservation of vibration and positional sensations and the presence of pain, numbness, and the loss of temperature sensation; and large fiber neuropathy, on the other hand, is characterized by muscle weakness, loss of vibration and position senses, and the lack of deep tendon reflexes. Foot drop is common.

- Some of the signs and symptoms of Autonomic Neuropathy include nausea and vomiting as the result of gastroparesis, orthostatic hypotension, tachycardia, constipation, diarrhea and dumping syndrome, urinary and fecal incontinence, diminished vaginal lubrication, erectile dysfunction and urinary retention

- Radiculopathies lead to pain, weakness and atrophy of the lower extremities. Thoracic polyradiculopathy leads to abdominal pain.

- Cranial Neuropathy: When the neuropathy affects the 3rd cranial nerve, known as the oculomotor nerve, these neuropathies can lead to diplopia, or double vision, ptosis, or drooping of the upper eyelid, and anisocoria, which is an unequal pupil size. Motor dysfunction occurs when the cranial neuropathy affects the 4th and/or the 6th cranial nerve(s.)

Treatment

When possible, the underlying cause, such as hyperglycemia, should be controlled and managed. Other treatments include symptomatic relief and the prevention of any complications. For example, symmetric polyneuropathy treatment includes pain management (topical capsaicin cream), the control of the blood glucose, and medications such as tricyclic antidepressants like imipramine and anticonvulsants like Neurontin (gabapentin), as indicated by the severity of this disorder. Proper turning and positioning prevents foot drop and other contractions relating to large fiber neuropathy.

Possible Nursing Diagnoses

- Pain r/t neuropathy and paresthesia
- Altered sensory functioning r/t neuropathy

Seizures

Seizures are caused by abnormal electrical activity in the brain. Seizures can be an acute primary event or the result of a cerebral trauma or insult such as stroke. The phases of seizure activity are the tonic phase, which is marked with excessive muscle tone, involuntary muscular contractions, a loss of consciousness, apnea and signs of autonomic nervous system dysfunction; and the clonic phase, which is characterized by alternating relaxation and muscular contraction. Oxygen and energy demands are greatly increased during a seizure. For example, cerebral energy demands and cerebral blood flow demands both increase by about 250%.

Epileptic seizures are classified as partial, or focal, seizures, which are further classified as simple partial and complex partial seizures and generalized seizures as determined by the presence or absence of a loss of consciousness. Generalized seizures are also subcategorized as generalized tonic-clonic seizures and non-convulsive seizures.

Some of the risk factors associated with seizures include hypoglycemia, cerebral tumors, brain infections, hypertension, renal or hepatic failure, and stress, among other things.

Signs and Symptoms

The signs and symptoms of seizures vary according to the specific type of seizure. Some of these signs and symptoms include loss of consciousness, a loss of responsiveness, cyanosis, apnea, pupil dilation, a lack of papillary responses to light, rhythmic periods of muscular contraction and muscular relaxation, tachycardia, profuse diaphoresis, increase salivation, hyperventilation, eye rolling, drooped or twitching lips, loss of bladder and/or bowel control and a blank trance-like stare, among other signs and symptoms.

Treatment

The goal of treatment is to address and remove the cause of the seizure(s.) The client should learn about the warning signs of a seizure, and to avoid factors that place them at risk for seizures. Clients should be encouraged to get and wear a medical emergency tag or bracelet that alerts others that they have a seizure disorder.

Acute treatment of seizures or status epilepticus involves the following:

- Clear the client's airway

- Diazepam 10 mg IV and repeat the dose after 15 minutes and 30 minutes if necessary, and if the client does not respond doubling the dose may be needed.

- Lorazepam 2-4 mg SL, SC or IV and repeat after 15 and thirty minutes if necessary

- Midazolam 5-10 mg SC or IV repeat after 15 minutes if necessary, and if the client does not respond doubling the dose may be necessary.

- Phenobarbital 100-200 mg SC or IV slowly over 30 minutes with 100 cc of saline. This also may need to be repeated.

Anticonvulsant medications that can be used to treat seizures are phenytoin 300 mg PO followed by 100-200 mg tid PO, carbamazepine 100 mg bid PO, Valproate 200 mg tid PO and lamotrigine, gabapentin and toprimate.

Corticosteroids, to decrease the edema around a mass, can be used to prevent and manage seizures that are secondary to brain metastasis.

Possible Nursing Diagnoses

- At risk for injury r/t seizures
- Altered level of consciousness r/t seizures

Extrapyramidal Symptoms

Clients who take antipsychotic medications are at greatest risk for extrapyramidal symptoms, although a few other medications can also place a client at risk.

Signs and Symptoms

Extrapyramidal symptoms can be categorized as dyskinesias, which are movement disorders, and dystonias which are disorders associated with muscular tension. Dyskinesias can be manifested with a number of involuntary, purposeless, repetitive movements including eye blinking, lip smacking, tongue thrusts, arm/leg/finger movements. Tardive dyskinesia symptoms, which occur after years of treatment with an antipsychotic drug, are likely to be permanent even after discontinuation of the antipsychotic drug.

Clients affected with akathisia have extreme inner or external restlessness, shakiness and jitters that can cause a complete inability to stay still, thus placing the client at risk for severe exhaustion. Tardive akathisia, like tardive dyskinesia, occurs with long-term medication use and it is often permanent and irreversible.

Dystonia is muscular contractions and twisting of body parts, particularly the neck. It can be very painful and it can affect all bodily parts. At times, the eyes are also affected. Tardive dystonia is often permanent after years of antipsychotic medication.

Other extrapyramidal symptoms mimic those of Parkinson's disease. For example, the client may be affected with strange finger and hand movements, a shuffling gait, uncontrollable speech and an inability to speak when the client is affected with vocal cord tics.

Treatment

Medication such as benztropine (Cogentin®) can be beneficial to the client to lessen these highly distressing symptoms. Additionally, the causative medication should be discontinued when the symptoms emerge in order to prevent permanent disability.

Possible Nursing Diagnoses

- Loss of self esteem r/t extrapyramidal symptoms
- At risk for communication problems r/t extrapyramidal symptoms (vocal tics)
- Pain r/t extrapyramidal symptoms

Paralysis

Paralysis is a symptom that can occur as the result of several causes including stroke, a spinal cord injury, autoimmune disorders like Guillain-Barre syndrome, polio, botulism, spina bifida, multiple sclerosis and nerve disorders such as amyotrophic lateral sclerosis (ALS), for example.

Signs and Symptoms

Spinal cord injuries can lead to quadriplegia, tetraplegia and paraplegia. Tetraplegia is the loss, or impairment of, sensory and/or motor function beginning at the cervical portion of the spinal cord. This type of injury causes diminished, or absent, functioning of the arms, trunk, pelvic organs and legs. Paraplegia, on the other hand, is the loss, or impairment of, sensory and/or motor function originating at the thoracic, lumbar or sacral portion of the spinal cord. This type of injury causes diminished, or absent, functioning of the trunk, pelvic organs and legs, while arm function remains normal.

Treatment

The treatment of paralysis depends on the cause and the symptoms. For example, reversible causes are corrected; disability is treated with restorative and rehabilitation care; and symptoms like pain are treated.

Possible Nursing Diagnoses

- Pain r/t paralysis
- Risk for disuse syndrome r/t paralysis
- Impaired mobility r/t neuromuscular impairment
- Powerlessness r/t self care as the result of paralysis

Spinal Cord Compression

The American Spinal Injury Association (ASIA)scale classifies spinal cord injuries from A to E, as based on sensory and motor function. For example, grade A spinal cord injuries are complete injuries and the most severe of all. There is no sensory or motor function whatsoever; grades B, C and D are incomplete injuries. Grade B consists of the lack of motor function at the level of the injury and below, and preserved sensory function. Grade C reflects the presence of motor function below the level of the injury, but the muscular function is impaired. Grade D, also an incomplete injury, has preserved motor function below the injury but the muscular function is not as severely impaired as it is for Grade C. Lastly, grade E reflects normal sensory and motor function.

Spinal cord injuries result from flexion, extension, compression and rotation forces. Flexion injuries occur most often as the result of an automobile accident when the head takes a blow with hyper-flexion of the spine; extension injuries occur when the head is tossed backwards; compression injuries can occur as the result of a fall, diving into shallow water and brain cancer. Vertebral bodies become compressed and wedged and shards of bone pierce the spinal cord with this type of injury. Lastly, rotational injuries lead to damage to the entire ligamentous structure; flexion rotation injuries are the most unstable of all types.

Signs and Symptoms

Initially, assess the ABCs (airway, breathing and circulation.) Respiratory dysfunction can occur when the diaphragm, intercostal muscles and accessory respiratory muscles are affected. Other possible signs and symptoms include impaired urinary function, paralysis, paralytic ileus, pain, particularly when the client has multiple traumas, nausea, vomiting, and hypothermia.

Treatment

Morphine or fentanyl is used for moderate to severe pain; other possible medications, as based on the particular client's spinal cord problem, can include anticonvulsants, tricyclic antidepressants, antiemetics and/or a nasogastric tube for nausea, vomiting and paralytic ileus, and the avoidance of cold intravenous fluids.

Respiratory and oxygenation needs are treated with BiPAP, mechanical ventilation and intubation, as indicated. Complications, such as deep vein thrombosis, are prevented with prophylactic anticoagulant therapy (low-molecular-weight heparin or low-dose heparin), compression stockings and intermittent sequential calf-compression. A urinary catheter is used to treat a contractile neuropathic bladder and to ensure adequate urinary output. Intake and output are monitored and accurately documented; and immobilization and stabilization are also essential aspects of care.

Possible Nursing Diagnoses

- At risk for respiratory compromise r/t spinal cord injury
- Loss of sensory function r/t spinal cord injury
- Impaired motor functioning r/t spinal cord injury

Increased Intracranial Pressure

The pressure within the cranial cavity is called intracranial pressure (ICP.) Intracranial pressure is affected with pressures from brain tissue, blood and cerebral spinal fluid. The normal ICP is from 5 to 15 mmHg. When the bony cranium is affected with increased pressure, it cannot be accommodated for. Increased intracranial pressure is life threatening. Cellular death and hypoxia occur.

The most common causes of increased intracranial pressure are cerebral, subarachnoid bleeding or hematoma, closed head trauma, a brain tumor, an infarction, a subdural or epidural hematoma, and brain infections.

Signs and Symptoms

Early signs of increased intracranial pressure include headache, diminishing level of consciousness, dilation of the pupils, slow pupil constriction, motor and/or sensory losses, and visual disturbances like kiplopia. Late signs and symptoms include hiccups, a fever, vomiting, decerebrate and/or decorticate posturing, and the other signs and symptoms associated with Cushing's reflex and Cheyne-Stokes respirations.

Cushing's reflex signs and symptoms are late signs of increased intracranial pressure, and they indicate severe brainstem ischemia. These signs and symptoms include hypertension, bradycardia, and a widening pulse pressure. Pulse pressure is the mathematical difference between the systolic and diastolic blood pressures. For example, the pulse pressure is 60 when a client's blood pressure is 120/60 (120-60= 60) and the pulse pressure will rise to 80 when the client's blood pressure changes to 160/80 (160-80=80.) This rise is referred to as a widening pulse pressure.

Cheyne-Stokes respirations have the classic signs of rapid, deep breathing with periods of apnea and abnormal posturing.

Decerebrate posturing, an abnormal body posture, consists of the arms and legs straight out, the toes pointed downward, and the neck and head arched backwards. The muscles are held very rigidly and tightly. Severe spasms of the back and neck (opisthotonos) may occur in severe cases. On occasion, the client may have decerebrate posturing on one side of the body and decorticate posturing on the other side of the body.

Decorticate posture, another abnormal posture, indicates severe brain damage. It is characterized by stiff bent arms turned towards the body, clenched fists held on the chest and straight stiff legs. This posturing indicates severe cerebral damage but it is typically not as pronounced as that manifested with decerebrate posturing.

Treatment

The goal of treatment, for some clients, is the preservation of life. Treatments vary according to the cause and the severity of the increased intracranial pressure. Surgical interventions are necessary in many cases, if the client chooses this option.

Medications that are used include intravenous osmotic diuretics, like mannitol, to remove fluid, corticosteroids to reduce edema, and anticonvulsant medications to prevent seizures.

A planned barbiturate coma is induced when there is a need to lower the metabolic demands of the brain and to prevent further brain damage. Additionally, artificial ventilation is often necessary and surgical interventions are sometimes indicated to eliminate the cause of the ICP.

Possible Nursing Diagnoses

- Confusion r/t increased intracranial pressure
- Pain r/t increased intracranial pressure
- Risk for alterations of breathing r/t increased intracranial pressure

CARDIOVASCULAR SYMPTOMS

Coagulation Problems

Coagulation problems result from the client's body being unable to effectively control blood clotting. There are a variety of different coagulation disorders, of which hemophilia is the most common. Other coagulation disorders include Christmas disease, which is also referred to as hemophilia B or Factor IX deficiency, disseminated intravascular coagulation, also known as consumption coagulopathy, thrombocytopenia, Von Willebrands disease, hypoprothrombinemia, factor XI deficiency which is also referred to as hemophilia C, and factor VII deficiency.

Signs and Symptoms

Depending on the individual disease or disorder, the signs and symptoms vary, but they include pain, severe bruising, coma, shortness of breath, shock and fatigue.

Treatment

Again, depending on the specific disease or disorder, the treatment varies. For example, for mild cases, medication can be used in order to stimulate the release of deficient clotting factors. In severe cases, the only way to stop the bleeding is by replacing the missing clotting factor with a transfusion.

Thrombotic Thrombocytopenia Purpura

Thrombotic thrombocytopenia purpura, also known as thrombocytopenia, is a blood disorder that forms clots in vessels all over the body.

Risk Factors

The risk factors include chemotherapy, estrogen and other hormone therapies, bone marrow transplantation and several types of cancer.

Signs and Symptoms

The signs and symptoms of thrombotic thrombocytopenia purpura include fatigue, pallor, headache, fever, confusion, altered level of consciousness, shortness of breath, tachycardia, jaundice, purpura and bleeding into the skin or mucus membranes.

Treatment

Treatments include plasma exchange to remove the antibodies that are affecting the blood and to replace clotting enzymes, a spleenectomy, and medications to suppress the immune system, such as corticosteroids or rituximab.

Nurses should assess and observe clients for the signs and symptoms of thrombotic thrombocytopenia purpura, particularly post operatively, when they have undergone bone marrow transplantation and/or they are taking chemotherapy, estrogen and other hormone therapies.

Related Nursing Diagnoses

- At risk for confusion and injury r/t thrombotic thrombocytopenia purpura
- Impaired cognitive functioning r/t thrombotic thrombocytopenia purpura

Disseminated Intravascular Coagulation (DIC)

This disorder occurs because of several underlying conditions and diseases. It does not occur as a primary condition. This disorder is unique and somewhat paradoxical. It affects thrombosis, or clotting, as well as bleeding. There is a lack of balance between anticoagulation and coagulation.

Risk Factors

Neoplastic acute leukemia, phoechromocytoma and adenocarcinoma are most often associated with disseminated intravascular coagulation. Some of the other risk factors associated with DIC, in addition to cancer, are hepatic disease, hypoxia, infections, especially gram negative sepsis, hypersensitivity reactions, and vascular disorders.

Signs and Symptoms

The chronic form of disseminated intravascular coagulation has a slow onset over weeks or months and it leads to excessive clotting without bleeding. Acute DIC occurs rapidly and it is marked with excessive clotting and then severe bleeding.

Other signs and symptoms can include headache, tachycardia, hypotension, changes in mood, behavior and/or level of consciousness, and peripheral cyanosis secondary to microvascular thrombosis.

Treatment

Non-pharmacological and pharmacological interventions aim to prevent life threatening complications, such as impaired perfusion and death, to maintain tissue and organ perfusion and the elimination of the root cause, if possible.

Specific interventions include the administration of blood products like packed red cells, and fresh frozen plasma to replace clotting factors and fluids. Hypoxia, acidosis, and hypotension are corrected and recombinant human activated protein C may be administered.

Nurses must closely assess for bleeding, fluid overload as the result of fluid/blood replacements, urinary and renal compromise. Hourly urine samples are collected to evaluate cardiac and renal perfusion and functioning.

Related Nursing Diagnoses

- Deficient fluid volume r/t hemorrhage and depleted clotting factors
- Impaired tissue perfusion r/t hypoxia and hypotension

Angina

Angina typically occurs as a result of atherosclerotic plaque buildup, plaque rupture, vasoconstriction, and the formation of a thrombus which may disrupt blood flow within the coronary artery in an intermittent manner.

Signs and Symptoms

The signs and symptoms of angina include chest pain or discomfort, which is described as squeezing pressure in the center of one's chest, and radiating pain to the arms, neck, jaw, shoulder or the back, nausea, fatigue, shortness of breath, sweating and dizziness.

Treatment

Treatment of angina includes lifestyle changes, such as smoking cessation, keeping fit, eating healthy, medications like nitroglycerine sublingually, angioplasty and stenting, or coronary bypass surgery. The ultimate aim of treatment is to reduce the symptoms and lower the risk for heart attack and death.

RESPIRATORY SYMPTOMS

Congestion

Chest congestion is an accumulation of mucous in the chest, which results from inflammation of the lower respiratory tract.

Signs and Symptoms

Signs and symptoms of chest congestion are easy to detect. These symptoms include coughing, wheezing, runny nose, labored breathing, chest pain, and shortness of breath.

Chest congestion can be a symptom of a disease or disorder like a flu, which also cause the client to experience fever, chills, malaise and body aches.

Treatment

Chest congestion can be treated with an antihistamine that contains diphenhydramine, and, if more serious and related to a bacterial infection, it can be treated with antibiotics. Some home remedies are inhaling steam and drinking hot tea and soup broth.

Related Nursing Diagnoses

- Alteration in respiratory status r/t congestion
- At risk for pulmonary infection r/t congestion

Cough

Coughing results from throat irritation.

Signs and Symptoms

Prolonged episodes of coughing can cause headaches, sleeplessness, urinary incontinence and broken ribs.

Treatment

A cough can simply be treated by an over-the-counter cough syrup and/or cough drops, but a more serious or severe cough, which can result from a disease or disorder ranging from strep throat to tuberculosis, lung cancer and a number of other disorders, may have to be treated with medications and treatments like bronchodilators and nebulizer treatments.

Related Nursing Diagnoses

- Rib pain r/t coughing

- Insomnia r/t coughing

Dyspnea

Dyspnea is shortness of breath, difficulty breathing, and labored breathing. Dyspnea is a symptom of a variety of different diseases and disorders.

Treatment

Immediate treatment for dyspnea includes providing the client with oxygen and the correction of the underlying causes, when possible. In extreme cases, intubation and mechanical ventilation may be necessary.

Related Nursing Diagnoses

- Fear and anxiety r/t dyspnea
- Inadequate oxygenation r/t dyspnea

Pleural Effusion

Pleural effusion is a collection of fluid in the pleural space around the lung. This is caused by excessive fluid production or a decrease in fluid absorption. A pleural effusion can occur in almost any type of cancer, but the most common causes of a malignant pleural effusion are lung and breast cancer. Pleural effusion can be the first sign of cancer, a reoccurrence of cancer or advanced stages of cancer.

Signs and Symptoms

Possible signs and symptoms include dyspnea, cough, chest pain and fever.

Treatment

The treatment of pleural effusion requires treating an underlying condition. For example, if bacterial pneumonia is present, the client can be given antibiotics. Drainage is often required if the pleural effusion is extensive, infected or inflamed. Other treatment methods include chest tubes to drainage and thoracentesis.

Related Nursing Diagnoses

- Dyspnea r/t pleural effusion
- Altered respiratory function r/t pleural effusion

Pneumothorax

A pneumothorax, or collapsed lung, occurs when there is a leakage of air into the area between the chest wall and the lungs. This abnormal collection of air leads to pressure on the lung, which can cause it to completely or partially collapse. A hemothorax has the same signs and symptoms as a pneumothorax, but a hemothorax occurs as the result of blood leaking into the area that occurs, for example, with trauma.

Signs and Symptoms

The signs and symptoms of a pneumothorax include chest pain and shortness of breath.

Treatment

Relieving pressure on the lung is the ultimate goal of treatment for a pneumothorax. Some cases, such as with a partially collapsed lung, the physician may choose to administer supplemental oxygen and monitor the client to see if the air is reabsorbed and the lung re-inflates. Cases that are more serious may require aspiration, chest tube placement to remove the air, and the surgical repair of the leaking area.

Related Nursing Diagnoses

- Chest pain r/t pneumothorax
- Dyspnea r/t pneumothorax

GASTROINTESTINAL SYMPTOMS

Constipation

Constipation is defined as fewer than three bowel movements a week that are hard and dry. It affects many palliative care and hospice clients as the result of immobility, dehydration, emotional stress, diminished food intake, the aging process, mechanical obstruction and medications such as opioids.

Constipation can be prevented at times when mobility, fluids, and a bowel regimen are initiated when the client will be taking opioids for pain.

Signs and Symptoms

Signs and symptoms of constipation include the following: excessive straining, painful, hard stools, abdominal fullness, nausea, vomiting and abdominal pain. A bowel obstruction can occur when constipation is not prevented and/or not treated.

Treatment

Pharmacological interventions include bulk additives, suppositories and enemas; at times manual finger evacuation may be necessary to prevent impaction. Dietary increases of fiber, increased fluids and activity can prevent episodes of constipation.

During the client's final days and hours, treatment is not indicated because of the discomfort associated with these interventions.

Related Nursing Diagnoses

- Constipation r/t immobility and low fiber diet
- Constipation r/t analgesic medications
- Abdominal pain and distention r/t constipation

Diarrhea

Diarrhea is loose, watery stools that occur on a frequent basis. Episodes of diarrhea can be acute and short-lived, and they can be long-term and the effect of a disease process such as a gastrointestinal infection and chronic disorders like Chron's disease and inflammatory bowel disease. Additionally, many medications can lead to diarrhea.

Signs and Symptoms

The signs and symptoms include frequent loose and watery stools, abdominal cramps and/or pain, fever, bloating, and bloody stools.

Treatment

Most of the time, diarrhea will pass on its own in a couple of days with the help of over-the-counter remedies.

Fluid and electrolyte balances must be monitored and maintained, particularly among the elderly, infants and young children. The client should attempt to maintain their fluid balance with dietary fluids. However, when this is not successful, intravenous fluids and electrolytes like potassium and sodium may be indicated.

Related Nursing Diagnoses

- At risk for fluid and electrolyte imbalances r/t diarrhea
- Abdominal cramping r/t diarrhea

Bowel Incontinence

Bowel incontinence, also known as fecal incontinence, is defined as the inability to control one's bowel movements, which then in turn cause stool or feces to leak out of the rectum unexpectedly and uncontrollably. This leakage can range from this slight leakage to a complete loss of bowel control.

There are several types of cancer, such as cancers to the anus and rectum, in which the client is more likely to experience diarrhea. It may be quite distressing and embarrassing to the client so the nursing staff must be sensitive to these feelings and always treat the client with respect and dignity.

Signs and Symptoms

In most cases bowel incontinence only occurs when a client is experiencing diarrhea, but there are cases of recurrent or chronic fecal incontinence.

Treatment

Bowel incontinence can be treated with anti-diarrheal drugs, laxatives and medications that slow down peristalsis. Adding fiber to the diet is also helpful since fiber adds bulk and solidity to the stool. If the bowel incontinence is linked to muscular damage, exercise to improve anal sphincter control as well as biofeedback, bowel training and sacral nerve stimulation may be indicated. Some surgical interventions are a sphincteroplasty, the correction of a rectal prolapsed and sphincter replacement.

Related Nursing Diagnoses

- At risk for skin breakdown r/t bowel incontinence
- Loss of self esteem r/t bowel incontinence

Ascites

Ascites is fluid built up in the area between the lining of the abdomen and the abdominal organs in the abdominal/ peritoneal cavity. Ascites is common among clients with malignancy, particularly cancer of the ovary, breast and those affecting the gastrointestinal tract, however, it is also found among palliative care clients affected with tuberculosis, heart failure and cirrhosis of the liver.

Signs and Symptoms

The client's abdomen becomes distended and uncomfortable and the client may have anorexia because the fluid is pressing on the stomach. Shortness of breath can occur when the fluid collection is pressing on the diaphragm. A dull sound is heard upon percussion, wave like abdominal movement are observed with the abdomen is percussed, and the abdominal skin becomes tight and taut with a flattened naval. Significant weight gains also occur. Acites can also lead to dependent swelling and edema.

Treatment

The conservative treatment for ascites includes a combination of a low-sodium diet and diuretics, such as furosemide, and careful monitoring of potassium and sodium serum electrolytes.

A therapeutic paracentesis is done to remove excessive fluid when diuretics are not helpful. This procedure is performed by inserting a needle into the space, with ultrasound guidance, to allow the evacuation of the excessive fluid. When the condition becomes chronic and recurring, a portosystemic shunt or a liver transplant may be indicated. These palliative, comfort measures, however, are not typically done during the final terminal phase of life, that is, hours to a few days before the cessation of life.

Related Nursing Diagnoses

- Shortness of breath and anorexia r/t ascites
- Alteration of bodily image r/t distended abdomen

Hiccups

Hiccups, also known as hiccoughs, singultus and synchronous diaphragmatic flutter, are involuntary contractions of the diaphragm, followed by a "hic" sound, which is caused by a sudden closure of one's vocal cords.

A large number of drug-induced or natural causes can cause hiccups. Gastrointestinal causes, such as gastroesophageal reflux disease and gastric distension, are the most frequent causes. Other causes include ascites, hepatic tumors, renal failure, hyponatremia, brain stem lesions, infections and medications such as the corticosteroids.

Signs and Symptoms

The only sign is the "hic" sound, although in some cases, the client feels a slight tightening sensation in their chest, abdomen or throat before the "hic" sound occurs.

Treatment

No treatment is necessary in most cases. If, however, the hiccups are caused by an underlying medical condition or a medication, the underlying condition should be treated. Hiccups that last for more than two days may require medications like chlorpromazine, which is an antipsychotic drug, metoclopramide (Reglan) which is an anti-nausea drug, or baclofen (Lioresal) which is a muscle relaxant.

Some nonpharmacological interventions include pharyngeal stimulation, rebreathing into a bag, and a nasogastric tube when severe and unrelenting. Multiple interventions, in combination, are often needed with unrelenting, intractable hiccoughs. These interventions include a pherenic nerve block and a surgically implanted device that delivers mild electrical stimulation to the client's vagus nerve.

Related Nursing Diagnoses

- Potential for impaired coping r/t unrelenting hiccups
- Potential for impaired communication and social interactions r/t unrelenting hiccups

Nausea and Vomiting

Nausea and vomiting are extremely common symptoms that can be caused by a wide variety of medications, diseases and disorders. For example, virtually all medications, especially narcotic analgesics, have nausea and vomiting as side effects; acute and chronic disorders along the life span including pregnancy's morning sickness and gastroenteritis are associated with nausea and vomiting; and, many illness and treatments like cancer and chemotherapy can also lead to these gastrointestinal side effects.

Signs and Symptoms

The most common signs and symptoms are abdominal discomfort, anorexia, the inability to retain food and water, fainting, blurred vision and signs of dehydration such as confusion, dark colored urine, poor urinary output, poor skin turgor, excessive thirst, dry mouth, dizziness, headaches, and sunken eyeballs, .

Treatment

Most cases of nausea and vomiting simply require rest, hydration, avoiding triggers such as foul smells, eating bland foods, and the use of over-the-counter medications for motion sickness. In more severe cases, antiemetics such as ondansetron, metclopramide, domperidone, and/or antinausea medications, such as zofran, phenegran, and emetrol can be used.

Related Nursing Diagnoses

- At risk for dehydration r/t nausea and vomiting
- Altered fluid and electrolyte imbalances r/t nausea and vomiting

Bowel Obstructions

In addition to tumors in the bowel, other risk factors associated with bowel obstructions are surgical adhesions, fecal impaction, gallstones, and the presence of foreign bodies, hematomas, strictures and congenital adhesive banding.

These obstructions can be mechanical and non-mechanical. They can also be complete or partial and incomplete. Mechanical obstructions occur as the result of adhesions, tumors, intussusceptions, gallstones, volvulus, which is intestinal twisting, hernias, fecal impactions and strictures. Non-mechanical obstructions occur as the result of diminished peristalsis, which can occur with Hirschsprung's and Parkinson's disease.

Waste products and bowel contents accumulate above the obstruction regardless of the cause. This leads to bowel edema and increased capillary permeability both of which lead to fluid and electrolyte imbalances because the plasma seeps into peritoneal spaces.

Signs and Symptoms

Bowel obstructions lead to increased capillary permeability and bowel edema. These changes lead to impaired fluid and electrolyte balances, vomiting, pain, rigidity, hypotension, tachycardia and fever. Severe complications include bowel gangrene, strangulation, third spacing of fluids, impaired renal perfusion and oliguria.

The table below summarizes the signs and symptoms of large and small intestinal bowel obstructions:

Signs and Symptoms	Small Intestine	Large Intestine
Abdominal Distention	Minimal	Greater distention

| Vomiting | Copious and frequent | Rare |

Bowel Movements	Less constipation	Pronounced constipation
Pain	Intermittent, cramping colicky pain	Low degree of cramping
Onset	Rapid onset	Gradual onset

Treatment

Intravenous fluids and electrolytes are used to treat any fluid and electrolyte imbalances; a nasogastric tube for suction is used to decompress the bowel; and antibiotics are sometimes used to prevent infection. Surgical interventions, typically done endoscopically, can eliminate adhesions. Additionally, a bowel resection with reanastomosis and a temporary colostomy may be indicated.

Related Nursing Diagnoses

- Pain r/t bowel obstruction
- Alteration of fluid and electrolyte balances r/t bowel obstruction

Gastrointestinal Bleeding

Gastrointestinal (GI) bleeding indicates pathology of any one or more gastrointestinal organs including the rectum, stomach, esophagus, small intestine, large intestine, colon, and anus. Lower GI bleeding occurs in the large intestine, rectum, or anus. Upper GI bleeding is bleeding in the esophagus, stomach, or small intestine.

Peptic ulcers are the most common cause of upper GI tract hemorrhage or bleeding, although this blceding can also result from a bacterial infection, esophageal varices and Mallory-Weiss tears, which are tears in the esophageal wall.

Colitis is the most common cause of lower gastrointestinal bleeding, but other disorders like Chiron's disease, food poisoning, a parasitic invasion, hemorrhoids and infections can cause a lower GI bleed or hemorrhage.

Signs and Symptoms

The signs and symptoms of GI bleeding can vary. For example, a dark, black tarry stool is a sign of an upper GI bleed and bright red, bloody stool indicates a lower GI bleed. Some of the other common signs and symptoms include:

- Paleness
- Weakness
- Vomiting of blood (ashematemesis) or coffee ground-like material
- Shortness of breath

Treatment

The treatment for gastrointestinal bleeds includes the following: gastric lavage, gastric suctioning, blood replacement, medications and intravenous fluids.

Related Nursing Diagnoses

- At risk for hypovolemic shock r/t gastrointestinal bleeding
- Ineffective tissue perfusion r/t gastrointestinal bleeding

GENITOURINARY SYMPTOMS

Bladder Spasm

A bladder spasm is defined as a contraction of the bladder that causes an urge to urinate, which is often accompanied by pain.

Signs and Symptoms

The signs and symptoms include cramping pain, which can range from slight to extreme, and sometimes a burning sensation when urinating.

Treatment

Treatment of a bladder spasm includes the avoidance of spicy and hot foods and beverages, timed voiding every 1 ½ to 2 hours, Kegel's exercises to strengthen and relax the bladder as well as other pelvic floor muscles, medications like anticholinergics, alpha blockers and an antidepressant like tolterodine, the use of a TENS unit (transcutaneous electrical nerve stimulation) which provides mild electrical pulses to the bladder which increases blood flow and strengthens the bladder, and an electrical stimulation implant (Inter-Stim), which is similar to a TENS unit, but it is implanted under the skin and programmed to send mild electrical impulses

Related Nursing Diagnoses

- Pain r/t bladder spasms
- Dysuria r/t bladder spasms

Urinary Incontinence

Urinary incontinence is an involuntary leakage of urine and a loss of bladder control. This is more common in women, due to childbirth, the fact that females have a shorter urethra than men, and menopause. As a result, women often have stress incontinence, which is urinary leakage that occurs when the person coughs, sneezes, or laughs. Cognitive impairments, decreased mobility, urinary tract infections, cerebrovascular accidents, spinal cord injury or other diseases and disorders can also lead to urinary incontinence.

At the end stages of life, clients can often experience problems with urinary incontinence. If the amount of urinary output is minimal, absorbent pads or briefs can be used.

Signs and Symptoms

The signs and symptoms are slightly different for the different types of urinary incontinence, as below:

- Overflow incontinence: This type of incontinence occurs when the client is not able to fully empty their bladder during voiding as the result of a number of factors including weak bladder muscles, tumors that block urine flow, and constipation. It occurs most often among males.

- Functional incontinence: This type of incontinence occurs most frequently among those who have cognitive dysfunction or severe physical disease. Complete uncontrollable bladder emptying occurs.

- Stress incontinence: There is a small leakage of urine when the affected client coughs, laughs, or sneezes, which causes increased pressure in the abdomen. This type of incontinence results from weakened pelvic floor muscles.

- Urge incontinence: This form of incontinence occurs as the result of an overactive bladder secondary to some bladder nerve damage. The client is simply not able to get to the bathroom quick enough after the urge to urinate occurs.

Treatment

Managing urinary incontinence includes bladder training, which is also referred to as continence training, pelvic muscle exercises, maintaining skin integrity and using external urinary drainage devices and briefs. Whenever possible, indwelling urinary catheters should be avoided because they can lead to infections.

Related Nursing Diagnoses

- Functional urinary incontinence r/t cognitive impairment at the end of life
- At risk for skin breakdown r/t urinary incontinence
- At risk of falls r/t urinary incontinence

Urinary Retention

Urinary retention occurs when urine accumulates in the bladder and it causes bladder distention. It occurs when the client is not able to empty their bladder completely and 200 to 250 ml, or 10% of the bladder capacity, is retained. Some of the conditions associated with urinary retention include prostate cancer, benign prostatic hypertrophy, a urethral tumor, other forms of obstruction and muscular dysfunction.

Signs and Symptoms

Clients with acute urinary retention can experience pain or discomfort, an urge to urinate with no urinary output, abdominal bloating, a weak flow of urine, and urinary leakage between voiding.

Treatment

Some interventions include maintaining adequate fluid intake and maintaining normal voiding habits. If these actions are not successful, a cholinergic drug to stimulate bladder contractions and to facilitate more complete bladder emptying can be used. Crede massage is used if the client has a flaccid bladder. This massage includes the manual pressing on the bladder.

Urinary catheterization for residual urine may be used, as well as an indwelling urinary catheter, however, whenever possible, catheterization should be avoided in order to prevent urinary tract infections.

Related Nursing Diagnoses

- Upper urinary tract distress r/t urinary retention
- Abdominal bloating r/t urinary retention

Urinary Bleeding (Hematuria)

Hematuria, or blood in the urine, can result from a number of disorders and conditions such as a urinary tract infections, aspirin use, bladder cancer, glomerulonephritis, renal cancer and trauma to the urinary tract.

Signs and Symptoms

Hematuria is visible as bright red to pink tinged urine (gross hematuria) but most often, it is discovered with urine laboratory testing. Hematuria can be asymptomatic or symptomatic with pain dependent on the cause of the hematuria.

Treatment

Treatment specifically for hematuria does not exist; however, the cause of the hematuria can often be corrected.

Related Nursing Diagnoses

- Fear r/t visible hematuria
- At risk for hypovolemic shock r/t urinary tract hemorrhage

MUSCULOSKELETAL SYMPTOMS

Impaired Mobility and Complications

The old advice, "Take an aspirin and go to bed," could not be further from good advice. Immobility leads to severe consequences in terms of many bodily functions and structures.

These hazards are described below:

- *The Musculoskeletal System*

    Some adverse musculoskeletal system effects of immobility include muscle weakness, muscular atrophy, contractures, stiff and painful joints and disuse osteoporosis.

- *The Respiratory System*

    Some adverse respiratory system effects relating to immobility include hypostatic pneumonia as the result of pooled respiratory secretions, atelectasis that is also the result of pooled secretions in the bronchiole, decreased respiratory movement, decreased vital capacity and shallow respirations.

- *The Circulatory System*

    Some of the physiological changes that occur as the result of immobility include diminished cardiac reserve, orthostatic hypotension that can place the person at risk for falls, venous stasis and venous vasodilation which can lead to the formation of emboli, dependent edema, thrombophlebitis and an increased use of the Valsalva maneuver.

- *The Urinary System*

    The urinary system is affected by urinary stasis, renal stones, or calculi, urinary retention, urinary incontinence and urinary tract infections.

- *The Integumentary System*

    Immobility places clients at risk for skin breakdown, pressure ulcers, and poor skin turgor.

- *The Metabolic System*

    Some of the complications of immobility relating to the metabolic system include a diminished metabolic rate, a negative nitrogen balance caused by an increased catabolic protein breakdown, anorexia and a negative calcium balance that is caused by the loss of calcium from the bones.

- *The Gastrointestinal System*

    Constipation and dry, difficult to evacuate stools are the result of immobility.

- *The Psychological and Neurological Systems*

    Some of the psychological hazards of immobility include a lowered mood, frustration and depression.

Related Nursing Diagnoses

- At risk for pressure ulcers r/t immobility
- Muscular weakness r/t immobility

Pathological Fractures

Pathological fractures occur when normal weight bearing and/ or normal use exceeds the ability of the bone to support the normal stress of the weight or movement.

Some of the risk factors for pathological fractures include high-risk occupations like tree cutting, some metabolic disorders, low bone density, and some degenerative diseases like osteoporosis and neoplastic disease.

Signs and Symptoms

Like other skeletal fractures, some of the signs and symptoms of pathological fractures include pain, muscle spasms, numbness, swelling, abnormal skeletal bone angulation and/or rotation, neurological impairment and distal ischemia, which are characterized by the Six Ps of:

1. Pallor (circulatory compromise)
2. Paresthesia (nerve pressure)
3. Pain (ischemia)
4. Polar coolness
5. Paralysis
6. Pulselessness (impaired arterial perfusion)

Treatment

Treatments include immobilization, fixation, pain management and the prevention of complications relating to skeletal fractures.

Pain management is accomplished with elevation of the affected body part, cool packs, analgesic medications, and immobilization of the affected limb, which relieves and prevents painful muscular spasms. Immobilization can consist of either external or internal fixation. Internal fixation is a surgical form of immobilization that utilizes pins, screws, rods, plates, bone grafts (autogenous grafts and allografts) or a total joint replacement such as a hip or knee replacement. External fixation is done with traction (Russell and Buck's traction), casts and braces such as a Halo brace.

Treatment also includes the prevention of complications and the treatment of complications, should they arise. Some of these complications include compartment syndrome secondary to casting, fat emboli, infections with open fractures, fracture blisters, deep vein thrombosis, osteomyelitis, post traumatic arthritis, delayed union, nonunion, necrosis, shock, as the result of blood loss, pain and temporary or permanent disability.

Related Nursing Diagnoses

- Impaired physical mobility r/t fracture
- Pain r/t fracture
- At risk for the impairment of skin integrity r/t immobility

Deconditioning and Activity Intolerance

Activity intolerance is defined as the lack of psychological or physical abilities to endure and to complete one's desired activities. Some of the factors that impair a client's activity tolerance are pain, general weakness, prolonged periods of bed rest, immobility and an inadequate oxygen supply. Among palliative care clients, deconditioning leads to activity intolerance. For example, muscular weakness may occur with prolonged bed rest and immobility; and the client's stamina, endurance and cardiovascular status may be compromised by their disease process and other factors.

Signs and Symptoms

The signs and symptoms of activity intolerance, in addition to the lack of ability to perform activities, are fatigue, complaints of weakness, dyspnea with activities, and an abnormal pulse rate and/or blood pressure during exertion and the performance of activities.

Treatment

Again, the treatment varies according to the cause. For example, psychologically depressed clients experiencing activity intolerance may benefit from psychological support, encouragement and motivational strategies. Cardiovascular alterations can be treated with medications and progressively increasing the person's activity; and cardiovascular deconditioning can be prevented and improved by placing the client's head of the bed up in an upright position several times a day. Additionally, muscular weakness can be improved with a planned exercise routine, range of motion exercises and the help of a physical therapist.

Related Nursing Diagnoses

- Excessive fatigue r/t deconditioning
- Anxiety r/t activity intolerance r/t activity intolerance
- Respiratory and cardiovascular alterations r/t deconditioning

SKIN AND MUCOUS MEMBRANE SYMPTOMS

Dry Mouth (Xerostomia)

Dry mouth, which is also referred to as xerostomia, is a condition in which the client's mouth is unusually dry. This can affect the client's ability to enjoy their food and also affects the health of their teeth. Saliva helps to prevent tooth decay by limiting bacterial growth as well as washing away any food particles left behind. So, if there is a lack of sufficient saliva, the health of the client's teeth is at risk. The enzymes in saliva also aid in digestion, therefore, a lack of saliva decreases a client's ability to fully digest their food.

Signs and Symptoms

The signs and symptoms of dry mouth include cracked lips, bad breath, sore throat, dryness in the mouth, thick and stringy saliva, split or sore skin at the corners of one's mouth, difficulty swallowing and speaking, a fungal infection in one's mouth, an altered sense of taste, and an increase in plaque, tooth decay and gum disease.

Treatment

If the cause of the client's dry mouth is the result of a specific medication, the physician may opt to adjust the client's dosage or switch them to another medication. There are also medications that can be helpful, such as pilocarpine (Salagen) or cevimeline (Evoxac), to stimulate the production of saliva, in addition to over-the-counter products and prescription products like Biotene and Therabreath that can help to eliminate dry mouth.

Related Nursing Diagnoses

- At risk for dental caries r/t dry mouth
- Loss of appetite r/t dry mouth and the loss of the taste sensation

Oral and Esophageal Lesions

There are a variety of different oral lesions including candidiasis, recurrent herpes labialis, recurrent aphthous stomatitis, erythema migrans, hairy tongue, and lichen planus.

Oral candidiasis can be seen as pseudomembranous candidiasis, glossitis, or perlèche (angular cheilitis.) In adults, this type of lesion can indicate an immune deficiency or another illness. A typically mild and self-limiting type of these lesions is herpes labialis.

Although normally a mild condition, recurrent aphthous stomatitis arises as the result of nutritional deficiencies, autoimmune disorders, and HIV. A waxing and waning disorder known as erythema migrans is a disorder with no known etiology.

Hairy tongue is a disorder that commonly is found among heavy smokers. It presents as elongation and hypertrophy of the filiform papillae and lastly, a chronic inflammatory condition known as oral lichen may be reticular or erosive.

These oral lesions all have risk factors, which include poor oral hygiene, age, tobacco use, alcohol consumption, and some systemic conditions.

Esophageal Varices

Esophageal variances occur when the veins in the lower part of the esophagus are abnormally enlarged under pressure (portal hypertension.) These are often seen in clients who have serious liver disease. These varices develop when scar tissue forms in the liver and a clot obstructs the normal blood flow to the liver. The blood flow into smaller vessels is unable to handle large volume of blood flow so the leaking of blood or even rupture and massive bleeding can occur. Rupture of the esophageal varices is an emergency life threatening situation.

Related Nursing Diagnoses

- At risk for hemorrhage r/t esophageal varices
- Abdominal distention r/t portal hypertension

Pruritus

Clients over the age of seventy, particularly those at the end of life, will experience this sensation.

Signs and Symptoms

Pruritus is an unpleasant cutaneous itching sensation that causes the client to feel the need to scratch. Pruritus can result from dry skin, some medications, and other causes.

Treatment

Treatments include avoiding hot or spicy foods, keeping the client cool, tepid baths or showers, careful drying, and applying a moisturizer afterwards can also help to alleviate some of the discomfort. In some cases, topical steroid ointments are used.

Related Nursing Diagnoses
- Discomfort r/t pruritus
- Cutaneous bleeding r/t scratching

Wounds, including Pressure Ulcers

Pressure sores have a variety of names associated with them, such as decubitus ulcers, trophic ulcers, stasis ulcers, ischemic ulcers and bedsores. These ulcers occur as the result of external forces such as pressure over a bony prominence of the body, moisture (incontinence), and shearing and friction when a client is pulled up and/or repositioned in the bed. Most pressure ulcers can be prevented.

Some of the intrinsic factors that place clients at risk for pressure ulcers are poor nutritional status, a thin person body type, a condition that prohibits a client's free movement (paralysis), some diseases like diabetes, vascular deficiencies, and incontinence.

The four stages of pressure sore development are as follows:

- Stage 1 consists of red skin that does not return to normal color after the pressure is relieved. There may also be tenderness or a burning sensation of the skin, and the skin area may also be edematous.

- Stage 2 is characterized by blistering, peeling and/or cracking of the skin.

- Stage 3 occurs when the full thickness of the skin and subcutaneous tissue damage occur. A serous bloodstained discharge is commonly evident at this stage. Slough, which is composed of dead tissue, forms and it appears as a black necrotic area and, at this stage, there is an invasion of rapid multiplying microorganisms as well.

- During Stage 4, as the full thickness of skin and subcutaneous tissue is destroyed, a deep ulcer is formed. There is exposure and possible damage to structures, such as fascia, muscle, connective tissue and bone underlying the ulcer.

Treatment

Prevention is the best cure. When pressure sores do develop, the goals of treatment are removing pressure from the affected area, treating any predisposing factors and the promotion of healing.

Related Nursing Diagnoses

- At risk for infection r/t loss of skin integrity
- At risk for pressure ulcers r/t immobility or poor nutritional status

PSYCHOSOCIAL, EMOTIONAL AND SPIRITUAL ISSUES

Some of the most commonly occurring psychological and emotional alterations associated with terminal diseases include anger, denial, grief and loss, fear and anxiety, guilt, depression, suicidal and homicidal ideation, loss of hope and meaning, sleep disturbances, alterations of bodily image, loss of control, poor coping, intimacy and relationship issues and nearing death awareness.

Anger and Hostility

Many clients in pain and/or at the end of life experience anger and hostility. Client's family members and significant others may also experience these same feelings. Anger is a common psychological response to these conditions, as described below in the Stages of Grieving model Kubler-Ross.

Simply defined, anger is a psychological or emotional state that is related to displeasure. It is often accompanied with feelings of guilt because it is not socially acceptable to be angry and to express these feelings. Outward expressions of anger can include hostility towards others, destructiveness, aggression and even violence.

Signs and Symptoms

At times, anger and hostility can be directed toward the precipitating event and at times it can be displaced toward others when the person employs the psychological defense mechanism of displacement. For example, a client who becomes angry about their loss of independence and functioning as a result of their illness and then directs this anger towards their spouse, family members, nurse and other members of the healthcare team, is using displacement.

Treatment

Nurses can intervene in terms of anger and hostility by accepting the fact that the client has the right to be angry and attempt to understand the meaning and the source of the anger. The nurse should also encourage the client to openly ventilate their anger.

Related Nursing Diagnoses

- Anger r/t situational crisis
- Fear r/t terminal illness

Anxiety

The North American Nursing Diagnosis Association (NANDA) defines anxiety as feelings of dread, discomfort, and apprehension. Anxiety leads to autonomic responses and the anticipation of danger.

Anxiety can be categorized as mild, moderate, severe and at panic level. Anxiety can also be further classified as death anxiety. This anxiety commonly affects those with terminal illnesses like cancer. Death anxiety is characterized by various degrees of dread and discomfort. The client may express fears about the events surrounding death like incontinence and the loss of cognitive abilities, fears about pain at the time of death, uncertainty regarding encountering a higher power, and fears about the impact of their death on family members, among other things.

Signs and Symptoms

The signs and symptoms of anxiety include affective ones (increased helplessness, irritability, fright and worry), behavioral ones (insomnia and vigilance), sympathetic ones (anorexia, increased pulse, blood pressure and pulse), physiological ones (diaphoresis and trembling), parasympathetic effects (fatigue, urinary changes, weakness and faintness) and cognitive changes (poor problem solving skills and a lack of an adequate attention span.)

Treatment

The nurse should assess the level of anxiety for both the client and the significant other. As based on this assessment, some of the treatments can include empathy when the anxiety is rationale, encouraging the person to ventilate their feelings and perceptions, explaining all procedures, and using some techniques like cognitive/behavioral therapy, relaxation techniques, positive self talk, massage and therapeutic touch.

Related Nursing Diagnoses

- Anxiety r/t situational crisis
- Death anxiety r/t terminal disease

Denial

Denial is a psychological defense mechanism. Psychological defense mechanisms, also referred to as ego defense mechanisms, are unconscious mechanisms that protect the client from stress and anxiety that can arise from inner tensions and conflicts. They are the precursor to coping in a cognitive, conscious manner.

Signs and Symptoms

Denial occurs when the client refuses to acknowledge any facts or realities that are threatening to them. It protects the person from being adversely affected with a traumatic event or reality until they are ready to do so. Denial often occurs when a client is diagnosed with a terminal disease like cancer and HIV/AIDS.

Some other psychological defense mechanisms, their purposes and some examples are below.

- Defense Mechanism: Reaction Formation

    Mechanism: The person acts out in a manner that is the opposite of what their true feelings are.
    Protective Purpose: Allows the person to act out their feelings in a more appropriate manner.
    Example: A spouse who resents their husband may support all of their ideas and suggestions in a cooperative and polite manner.

- Defense Mechanism: Sublimation

    Mechanism: A socially unacceptable sexual or aggressive urge is replaced with a socially acceptable activity that substitutes for this urge.
    Protective Purpose: This defense mechanism protects the person from acting in a socially unacceptable, impulsive manner.
    Example: A person with incestuous feelings may become active in a church.

- Defense Mechanism: Undoing

    Mechanism: Undoing allows the client to feel as though they have made up for, and atoned, for wrongdoing.
    Protective Purpose: This allows the person to rid themselves of guilt by atonement for one's wrongdoings.
    Example: An abusive husband brings flowers home to his wife.

- Defense Mechanism: Compensation

    Mechanism: Personal weakness is covered up with overachievement in another area.
    Protective Purpose: This ego defense mechanism allows the person to protect their ego and level of self-esteem by excelling in another area to make up for their weakness.
    Example: A young child, who cannot excel in school like his older sibling, may choose to play a piano, and excel in it, to make up for his scholastic weaknesses.

- Defense Mechanism: Displacement

    Mechanism: Displacement moves hostility from one person, or object, to another person, or object.
    Protective Purpose: The purpose of this defense mechanism is to allow the affected individual to express their feelings, but in a manner that is less harmful and dangerous to other people, or objects.
    Example: A man who has been fired from work may come home and punch a hole in the wall, rather than punching the boss in the face.

- Defense Mechanism: Projection

    Mechanism: The client blames other people and/or the environment for the client's weaknesses, shortcomings, and failures.
    Protective Purpose: This defense mechanism helps the client to protect their own self-image and self-esteem by placing blame on other people or the environment.
    Example: A college student who fails out of college blames the college and the professors rather than self.

- Defense Mechanism: Repression

    Mechanism: Repression helps the person to keep threatening thoughts, desires and feelings deep down so they do not erupt into consciousness.
    Protective Purpose: This ego defense mechanism protects the person from trauma until they are ready to cope and deal with it.
    Example: A client may experience repressive amnesia after a traumatic automobile accident which does not allow them to remember any events surrounding and after the accident.

- Defense Mechanism: Regression

    Mechanism: Regression helps the person to a less demanding and threatening stage of development.
    Protective Purpose: This ego defense mechanism allows the person to move back to a previous stage of development when they were cared for and dependent upon others.
    Example: An ill hospitalized 8-year-old child may regress to thumb sucking and bed-wetting.

- Defense Mechanism: Identification

    Mechanism: The affected client imitates the behaviors of a person that they fear.
    Protective Purpose: This defense mechanism helps the client to preserve the value of self and to prevent personal devaluation.
    Example: A child imitates the father that she fears.

- Defense Mechanism: Minimization

    Mechanism: The affected client minimizes the significance of a problem.
    Protective Purpose: This mechanism allows the person to avoid taking responsibility and accountability for their own actions.
    Example: A diabetic client with severe leg ulcerations may state that it is "no big deal."

- Defense Mechanism: Rationalization

    Mechanism: Attaching socially acceptable motives and faulty logic to actions and behaviors.
    Protective Purpose: This helps the person to cope with their inability to meet standards and goals.
    Example: A husband who pushes his wife rationalizes it by stating that his wife was not hurt.

- Defense Mechanism: Introjection

    Mechanism: A person accepts the norms, values and beliefs as one's own despite the fact that they are not consistent with, and often contrary to, those that the person previously held.
    Protective Purpose: This ego defense mechanism prevents the person from being ostracized by society.
    Example: A person may suddenly embark upon a healthy lifestyle and personal responsibility when, in the past, they did not.

- Defense Mechanism: Intellectualization

    Mechanism: Forced rational thinking is used to decrease the significance of a threatening and traumatic event.
    Protective Purpose: Intellectualization protects the person from psychological trauma and pain.
    Example: The spouse of a diabetic who has died may state that her husband did not want to live any longer with his complications of diabetes.

Treatment

The nurse should not strip these mechanisms away from the client. The nurse should simply acknowledge the person and their feelings but NOT argue with the client about their lack of insight or better coping mechanisms. These mechanisms are beneficial to the client; they protect the person from psychological distress and other psychological problems.

Related Nursing Diagnoses

- Ineffective coping r/t denial
- Denial r/t situational crisis

Depression

Depression, of varying degrees, often affects the client and those close to the client when the person is affected with a serious, terminal illness like cancer. Depression leads to physical, emotional and cognitive changes.

Signs and Symptoms

The signs and symptoms of depression include feelings of hopelessness, helplessness, sadness, dejection, despair, sleep loss, listlessness, headache, weight loss, anorexia, social withdrawal, lack of sexual desire, crying, poor levels of concentration, poor decision making and problem solving skills, diminished performance, personality changes, and a lack of self-worth and self-esteem.

Treatment

The care and treatment for a depressed client is multifaceted. The client needs social support, perhaps spiritual support, cognitive behavioral therapy, and often medications such as antidepressants, and nonpharmacological approaches such as stress reduction and relaxation techniques.

Related Nursing Diagnoses

- At risk for depression r/t terminal disease
- Chronic sorrow r/t unresolved grief
- Hopelessness and helplessness r/t depression

Fear

Fear is a feeling of dread and apprehension relating to some impending danger or threat. It can result from a real or unreal thereat, but, nonetheless, the client is adversely affected with it. Although fear and anxiety are highly similar and often occur simultaneously, they are also different. Fear is typically related to a current threat and anxiety is most often related to a future, anticipated threat. Lastly, anxiety is vaguer than fear; anxiety often arises from emotional conflict and fear is most often associated with a specific physical or psychological threat.

Signs and Symptoms

Some of the signs and symptoms include apprehension, muscular tension, feelings of dread, panic, terror, jitteriness, diminished cognition and problem solving skills, dyspnea, dry mouth, fatigue, rapid pulse and respirations, increased systolic blood pressure, nausea, vomiting, pallor, pupil dilation, increased alertness with a narrowed focus on the source of the fear, avoidance and/or aggression.

Treatment

Interventions, after assessment, can include confronting the fear, verbalizing the fearful feeling, assisting the client to distinguish between real and imagined treats, and psychological support measures such as cognitive behavior therapy, relaxation techniques and massage.

Related Nursing Diagnoses

- Diminished thought and problem solving processes r/t fear
- Ineffective coping r/t irrational fears
- Distress r/t fear

Distress

Distress can be described as troubling feelings that can range from mild to severe and even disabling. A client can experience distress at anytime from diagnosis to the end of life. Its intensity can vary and become more severe as the client's disease or disorder progresses. It can affect coping with even the least complex situations.

Signs and Symptoms

Distress can be seen with a variety of different physical, emotional, mental and behavioral symptoms, including back pain, neck pain, tension headaches, migraine headaches, muscle tension, dry mouth, enlarged pupils, diarrhea, constipation, moodiness, depression, anxiety, nightmares, forgetfulness, difficulty concentrating, racing thoughts, frustration, irritability, mumbled or fast speech, defensiveness, and nervous habits, such as biting nails, foot tapping, and an inability to sit still.

Treatment

The treatment for distress can include relaxation techniques, counseling, and the support of family, friends and healthcare personnel to overcome their feelings. Some of the symptoms can be treated with medications such as antidepressants, benzodiazepines, and pain medications, as indicated.

Related Nursing Diagnoses

- Physical pain r/t distress
- Ineffective coping r/t distress

Grief and Loss

Loss, often associated with grief, is multidimensional. Loss can be actual, perceived, or anticipated. It occurs when a person has a significant change that causes the loss of something of value, when the person anticipates a loss and when the person has a perceived the loss of something of value.

Grieving is a normal response that includes physical, emotional, spiritual, social and intellectual responses. Sources of loss can originate from many things including an intrapersonal loss of self and one's bodily image and extrapersonal losses like the loss of savings with the costs of medical care. All losses affect the client.

Perceived losses are those losses that are not verifiable by others. This perception, although faulty, still impacts on and affects the person. People have anticipatory grief and loss before an actual or perceived loss actually occurs. For example, a son may undergo severe anticipatory loss and grief soon after his mother has been diagnosed with terminal cancer. Similarly, a woman may have anticipatory loss relating to her their loss of sexuality after a mastectomy.

Clients and significant others are affected with grief and loss.

Theories and Conceptual Frameworks Relating to Grief and Loss

- Kubler Ross's Stages of Grieving

    Similar to the other theories of loss, grieving and death, Kubler Ross's stages of grieving includes:

    - Denial
    - Anger
    - Bargaining
    - Depression
    - Acceptance

    Bargaining is a unique phase of this theory. During the bargaining stage, the client negotiates and bargains to avoid the loss. Spiritual support is often helpful during this stage.

- *Engel's Stages of Grieving*

    According to Engel, the stages of grieving are as below:

    - Shock and disbelief
    - Developing awareness
    - Restitution
    - Resolving the loss
    - Idealization
    - Outcome

    During shock and disbelief the client denies the loss and refuses to accept it. Later the client consciously acknowledges the loss and may even express anger towards others including family members and healthcare professionals.

    During the resolution stage, the client contemplates the loss and may accept a dependent role in terms of their support network. Clients' family members may deify and idealize the lost loved one and may, also, experience guilt and ambivalence.

During the outcome phase of Engel's model, the person adjusts to the loss as based on the characteristics of the loss, as discussed above.

- *Sander's Phases of Bereavement*

The phases of bereavement, according to Sander's theory, are:

- Shock
- Awareness of the loss
- Conservation and withdrawal
- Healing or the turning point
- Renewal

These phases are quite similar to those of Engel with some variations. For example, during the conservation and withdrawal phase, the person will withdraw from others and attempt to restore their physical and emotional wellbeing; and during the healing stage, the person will move from emotional distress to the point where they are able to learn how to live without the loved one. During the renewal phase, the person is able to independently live without the loved one.

Signs and Symptoms

The defining characteristics of grief can include sleep disturbances, altered immune responses, anger, blame, withdrawal, pain, panic, distress, suffering and alterations with neuroendocrine functioning.

Treatment

Nurses can assist the client with the grieving process by encouraging the person to ventilate their feelings, by encouraging effective coping strategies, by involving the family and significant others in the care of the client, and, when needed, refer the client and significant others to sources of psychosocial and spiritual support.

Related Nursing Diagnoses

- Distress r/t grief and loss
- Anticipatory grieving r/t terminal illness
- At risk for complicated grief r/t the death of a loved one

Guilt

Like all of the other psychosocial issues, the family and significant others are often affected with feelings of guilt and ambivalence. For example, the client may experience feelings of guilt for the effect that their lung cancer is having on the family unit after years of the family's attempts to get the client to stop smoking. A client may also feel guilty about leaving their family in poor financial status because of the medical expenses associated with the illness. Families may also experience feelings of guilt because they may have not cared for the person enough or they are no longer able to care for the palliative care client in the home.

The purpose of guilt, when grounded in fact, is to alert the person that they have done some wrong. This feeling of guilt then encourages the person to change behavior so they no longer violate social and moral standards.

Signs and Symptoms

Some of the signs and symptoms associated with guilt can include physical, psychological and spiritual distress and despair.

Treatment

Nurses can teach the client about the purpose of guilt in terms of learning and changing behavior, encouraging the client to make amends, facilitating the client's acceptance of the fact that they did something wrong but there is a need to move on and grow, and to understand that humans are not perfect and that forgiveness is possible.

Clients and family members may need psychological, spiritual and religious support to resolve feelings of guilt.

Related Nursing Diagnoses

- Distress and despair r/t guilt
- Spiritual distress r/t guilt

Loss of Hope and Meaning

The loss of hope can have psychological and spiritual or religious meanings and sources. For example, a person who is depressed may have feelings of hopelessness and no view of the future. The same client may also experience a spiritual loss of hope.

Signs and Symptoms

A client who is experiencing a loss of hope experiences a subjective state in which the person sees few or no alternatives. This leads to their inability to garner the energy and motivation to act on their own behalf.

Some of the signs and symptoms include decreased appetite, passivity, withdrawal, flat affect, a lack of involvement in care and the lack of motivation and initiative.

Treatment

Some of the nursing interventions for clients experiencing loss of hope and meaning include monitoring the client for suicide risk, assisting the client to discover sources of hope, assisting with problem solving, decision making, goal setting and coping, and encouraging the client to verbalize their feelings in an open and trusting environment.

Related Nursing Diagnoses

- At risk for suicide r/t loss of hope
- Spiritual distress r/t loss of meaning
- Despair r/t the loss of hope and the loss of meaning

Nearing Death Awareness

Clients and family members have one of three types of awareness. Levels of awareness affect how the nurse communicates with these clients. The three types of awareness are closed awareness, mutual pretense and open awareness.

Closed awareness is defined as an unawareness of the impending death and terminal illness. Although not as often as was done in the past, some family members may choose to withhold complete and accurate information about the client's condition from the client affected with the illness. This poses ethical and communication challenges

Mutual pretense is the type of awareness that is typified when the client and significant others have an awareness of the client's condition but all, including the client, avoid all discussions about it. Mutual pretense leaves the affected client with no one to talk to about their fears and concerns because the client does not discuss things with the family and the family does not openly discuss things with the client.

Open awareness is the most beneficial of all levels of awareness for the client and their significant others. All know about the terminal nature of the disease and impending death and all are able to talk about it. Open awareness facilitates the client's finalization of plans and affairs, such as funeral arrangements.

Signs and Symptoms

The signs, symptoms and client/significant others' interaction depend on the level of awareness. For example, closed awareness is characterized by a lack of authentic communication and planning for the end of life; mutual pretense may lead the client to be depressed and feel alone; and open awareness is marked with beneficial family dynamics, realistic thinking, goal setting and final planning.

Treatment

Nurses can help the client and the family members to achieve open awareness within an open and trusting environment in which the client and family members are able to fully and openly express their fears and feelings.

Related Nursing Diagnoses

- Risk for ineffective family coping r/t dysfunctional levels of awareness
- Potential for open awareness r/t impending death

Sleep Disturbances

There are several factors that affect both the quantity and the quality of sleep. The quantity of sleep refers to total time a person sleeps; and the quality of sleep refers to how energetic and refreshed the person feels when they wake up.

Some of the factors that adversely affect a client's sleep and the quality of their sleep include pain, illness, respiratory dysfunction, physical and/or emotional distress, endocrine system disturbances like hypothyroidism which decreases stage IV sleep, some medications like steroids, narcotics, decongestants, bronchodilators, beta-blockers, antidepressants, and amphetamines, the physical environment (noise, lighting and room temperature), the lack of exercise, anxiety which stimulates the sympathetic nervous system and increases norepinephrine blood levels, and stimulants like caffeine and alcohol use.

Signs and Symptoms

There are a number of sleep disturbances or disorders that affect people. It is important for all nurses to be aware of them in order to help with their assessment of the client's sleep complaints and sleep/rest cycles.

Among the most common sleep disorders are insomnia, sleep apnea, and parasomnias. Insomnia is the most common sleep complaint in this country. Insomnia is an inability to fall asleep, a sleep induction disorder and/or to remain asleep, which is referred to as a sleep maintenance disorder. People with insomnia may experience irritability, problems concentrating, sleepiness during the daytime, and waking up when not feeling rested.

Sleep apnea is the cessation of a person's breathing that occurs frequently throughout the night. These periods of apnea can occur five, or more times, per night and the duration can last for longer than ten seconds every hour. The symptoms of sleep apnea include excessive daytime sleepiness, snoring, several sudden awakenings throughout the night, irritability, morning headaches, memory and cognitive problems and difficulties falling asleep.

The treatment for sleep apnea depends on the cause. For example if the apnea is related to enlarged tonsils the tonsils can be removed. Other treatments include the use of a CPAP device, laser removal of excessive tissue in the pharynx, and weight loss.

Parasomnias are different types of behaviors that can occur during sleep such as bruxism, which is clenching or grinding of the person's teeth, enuresis, which is bedwetting, sleepwalking, sleep talking and periodic limb movements that awaken the client.

Treatment

The promotion of sleep often depends on correcting the problem that causes the sleep disruption. The use of sleep medications should only be used as a last resort.

Some of the things to facilitate rest and sleep include pain relief, setting a regular bedtime and wake time, eliminating or decreasing nap times, avoiding exercise and stressful activities prior to bedtime, establishing a quiet, environmentally comfortable sleep environment that is conducive to sleep, and nonpharmacological nursing interventions such as massage and relaxation techniques.

Related Nursing Diagnoses

- Sleep deprivation r/t sleep disorder
- Sleep disturbance r/t anxiety and fear at the end of life

Suicidal and Homicidal Ideation

Most often a patient attempting suicide is depressed. This depression can be previously diagnosed or undiagnosed at the time of the suicide attempt.

Signs and Symptoms

Some of the most commonly occurring signs of suicide include lack of interest in the future, an overwhelming sense of guilt and/or shame, a significant drop in school or work performance, written or spoken notices of suicide intention, saying goodbye, dramatic changes in the personality or appearance, irrational, bizarre behavior, giving away possessions, putting affairs in order, changed eating or sleeping patterns, and self-harming actions, such as overdoses, which can be lethal to the person.

Even though confidentiality is both ethically mandated and legally required in most circumstances, confidentiality can legally and ethically be compromised when safety is at risk. For example, a nurse must report and disclose when a client tells the nurse that they plan on euthanizing their sick spouse and then committing suicide.

The assessment of a suicidal client includes data about the suicide plan, the client's degree of intent, the duration of the depression, factors that led to the depression, and information about the client's current feelings about suicide and death. For example, the nurse may ask the client about their thoughts about dying and/or living.

Like suicidal ideation among clients at the end of life, the same thoughts may affect family members and significant others. For example, an elderly woman may contemplate suicide because they just cannot accept the fact that she will be alone and without her husband.

Treatment

All threats of suicide must be taken seriously and not minimized. The primary intervention is prevention. It is vital that all healthcare personnel approach any and all suicidal or self-harming clients with caring, compassion and empathy. All interactions with these clients must be done in a non judgmental and supportive manner and all healthcare workers should remain calm, trusting and open with the client.

Open-ended questions, rather than judgmental closed-ended questions, should be employed during therapeutic communication with the suicidal client and clients should be encouraged to fully express their feelings. An example of an open-ended non-judgmental question that you could ask in order to assess the client's feelings is, "Tell me more about how you are feeling now."

The appropriate use of silence is also used in communication. Silence conveys caring, a willingness to listen, compassion, openness and interest in the client and what they are saying. A conversational and relaxed method of communication is used when communicating with a suicidal patient.

Constant observation and the use of restraints or seclusion may be necessary when the risk of suicide and self harm are high. The safety of the suicidal person is the MOST important initial intervention for a suicidal patient. For some suicidal patients, the ability to speak with someone and feel as though they are being listened to, understood and cared for may be all that is needed to resolve their crisis, particularly when the client has no previous history of a mental disorder.

Antidepressants are the most commonly prescribed medications for those at risk for suicide as a result of depression. Antipsychotic and anti anxiety medications are also used depending on the status of the client.

Related Nursing Diagnoses

- At risk for suicide r/t depression
- At risk for suicidal ideation r/t depression

Intimacy and Relationship Issues

Terminal illness and its physical and psychological effects can lead to several sexual changes in the client. These changes in sexuality vary according to the client, their illness and any treatments that they are taking. For example, a woman with breast cancer who is being treated with chemotherapy may have a decrease in libido, and a man with prostate cancer, who is being treated through radiation therapy, can experience no changes in libido, or sexual desire.

Signs and Symptoms

The National Cancer Institute (NCI) states that the loss of sexual desire, depression, anxiety, early menopause, body image alterations, pain during penetration, and erectile dysfunction can adversely affect patients and their sexuality.

Treatment

Patients who experience difficulties regarding their sexuality are encouraged to seek help from the nurse, and/or other professionals like a sex therapist or psychologist. Patients may also benefit from patient education about their changes in sexuality in terms of their problem, the common occurrence of this problem and ways that the client can cope with, and correct, their sexual concerns. Unfortunately, due to the stigma attached to sexual dysfunction and counseling for it, many patients may be too embarrassed to discuss their problems.

There are a variety of things, such as medications, surgery and assistive devices that can be helpful, depending on what problems the patients is experiencing. For example, an assistive device, such as a penile implant can be used for men with erectile dysfunction, lubricators and vaginal dilators can be used to help to ease the pain or discomfort a woman may be experiencing when they are having vaginal intercourse.

The National Cancer Institute recommends that couples discuss all their concerns and feelings about the current state of their sexual life and try to work together to find ways with which they can remain in a close and loving relationship, as they cope with, and adjust to, changes in sexuality.

Related Nursing Diagnoses

- At risk for sexual dysfunction r/t chemotherapy
- At risk for sexual dysfunction r/t radiation therapy
- At risk for sexual dysfunction r/t end of life symptoms

NUTRITIONAL AND METABOLIC SYMPTOMS

Anorexia

Dying clients often experience anorexia, or loss of appetite, and marked weight loss. It is often quite difficult for clients to accept the fact that they are dying so having the inability eat and/or drink can be very upsetting and distressing for the client and significant others.

Treatment

Intravenous fluids, total parenteral nutrition, and tube feedings can be used if the client chooses to have these treatments. When the client refuses these treatments, nurses and family members have to accept this choice.

Related Nursing Diagnoses

- Cachexia and wasting r/t anorexia
- Weakness r/t altered nutrition

Cachexia and Wasting

Cachexia, also referred to as wasting syndrome, occurs when a client loses both weight and muscle mass when they are not trying to do so. This syndrome is often seen in clients with cancer, HIV/AIDS, COPD, tuberculosis, congestive heart failure, failure to thrive, and many other serious diseases and disorders.

Signs and Symptoms

The three major symptoms associated with cachexia are diminished quality of life, substantial, unintentional weight loss, and a loss of appetite.

Treatment

The treatment of cachexia can be quite challenging. The ultimate goal of treatment is to increase anabolic processes, which build muscle, and to decrease the catabolic processes that result in muscle breakdown. The interventions typically include a combination of dietary changes, which includes the slow increase in caloric intake, nutritional supplements, such as fish oil, increased exercise, which can help to increase the client's appetite, and medications, such as testosterone, medical marijuana, Celebrex, Zyloprim and others depending on the client's needs.

Related Nursing Diagnoses

- Weakness r/t cachexia and muscle wasting
- Ineffective protection r/t inadequate nutrition

- Imbalanced nutrition; less than bodily requirements r/t a biological inability to an inability to ingest foods and fluids secondary to terminal disease

Dehydration

Dehydration occurs when one loses more fluid than is taken in. Fluid losses occur with normal bodily functions like urination, defecation, and perspiration and with abnormal physiological functions such as vomiting and diarrhea.

Dehydration can lead to serious physical and mental problems. Dehydration can be classified as mild, moderate and severe.

Signs and Symptoms

The signs and symptoms of mild to moderate dehydration are thirst, dry mouth and skin, constipation, headache, lightheadedness, dizziness, and decreased urinary output. The signs and symptoms of severe dehydration include confusion, the lack of diaphoresis, scant dark yellow or dark amber urine, anuria, sunken eyes, hypotension, tachycardia, tachypnea, fluid and electrolyte imbalances, dry skin that lacks good turgor, extreme thirst, a fever, delirium, confusion, unconsciousness and depressed fontanels in infants.

Treatment

The treatment for dehydration is rehydration. If the client is unable to orally replace fluids it may be necessary to replace the fluids intravenously.

Related Nursing Diagnoses

- Deficient fluid volume r/t fluid volume losses
- Impaired oral mucus membranes r/t decreased salivation
- At risk for renal impairment r/t dehydration
- Confusion r/t dehydration

Electrolyte Imbalances

Simply stated, electrolytes are minerals that carry an electrical charge. For example, sodium and potassium are positively charged electrolytes and chloride is a negatively charged electrolyte. The most common electrolytes are calcium, chloride, magnesium, phosphorous, potassium and sodium.

Electrolyte imbalances can occur as the result of many causes including vomiting, diarrhea and endocrine system alterations.

Signs and Symptoms

The signs and symptoms of deficient and excessive electrolytes vary greatly since different electrolytes perform different functions. Some of the signs and symptoms associated with imbalances of the most common electrolytes are shown below:

Electrolyte Imbalance and Normal Value	Description	Signs and Symptoms	Treatment	Related Nursing Diagnoses
Calcium: 8.5-10.6 mg/dL				
Hypercalcemia	High levels of calcium in the blood	Bone pain, muscular weakness, anorexia, nausea, vomiting, abdominal pain, cardiac arrhythmias, paresthesia, depression, weight loss and psychosis	Extensive intravenous fluid replacement, large doses of vitamins A and D, loop diuretics, decreased calcium intake, an increased fluid intake of 2 liters or more per day, and medications, such as zoledronate, alendronate or pamidronate

A surgical partial or complete removal of the parathyroid glands | At risk for pathological fractures r/t bone decalcification

Pain r/t skeletal bone decalcification |

| Hypocalcemia | Low levels of calcium in the blood | Dry scaly skin, brittle nails, coarse hair, muscle cramps in the back or legs, respiratory difficulties, cardiac arrhythmias and neurological or psychological symptoms such as hallucinations, memory loss, depression, delirium, seizures and confusion | Supplemental calcium and vitamin D to increase the absorption of calcium | Pain r/t hypocalcemia

At risk for alterations of respiratory and cardiovascular function r/t hypocalcemia |
|---|---|---|---|---|
| **Chloride**

96 to 106 mEq per liter | | | | |
| Hyperchloremia | High levels of chloride in the blood | Asymptomatic or dehydration, diarrhea, vomiting, high blood sugar, Kussmaul's breathing, dyspnea, intense thirst, weakness, tachypnea, hypertension, pitting edema, diminished cognitive ability and possible coma | Correction of the underlying cause, I.V. infusions of sodium bicarbonate or Lactated Ringer's | Alteration of the level of consciousness r/t hyperchloremia

Respiratory alterations r/t hyperchloremia |

Hypochloremia	Low levels of chloride in the blood	Muscle spasticity or tetany, shallow and/or depressed breathing, muscle weakness, hyponatremia, muscle twitching, sweating, and high fever	Hydration for the correction of underlying dehydration, electrolyte replacement and the consumption of potassium rich foods.	Pain r/t spasticity and tetany

Pyrexia r/t hyponatremia |
| **Magnesium**

1.2 to 2.5 mg/dL | | | | |
| Hypermagnesemia | High levels of magnesium in the blood | Generalized weakness, hypotension, cardiac arrhythmias, drowsiness, respiratory paralysis, CNS depression and coma | The cessation of magnesium containing drugs such as laxatives and antacids.

Calcium gluconate injection, dextrose, insulin, calcium chloride and renal dialysis. | Risk for alterations of respiratory and cardiovascular function r/t hypermagnesemia |
| Hypomagnesemia | Low levels of magnesium in the blood | Numbness, muscle weakness, muscle spasms or cramps, fatigue, convulsions and Nystagmus | Medications for symptomatic relief

Intravenous fluids and magnesium replacement | Pain r/t muscular spasms and cramps |

Phosphorous 2.4 - 4.1 mg/dL				
Hyperphosphatemia	High levels of phosphorous in the blood	Typically asymptomatic but it can lead to renal osteodystrophy, secondary hyperparathyroidism and ectopic calcification.	Treatment of the underlying cause; calcium carbonate tablets to bind to the phosphate	At risk for osseous tissue deposits in soft tissue and bodily organs r/t hyperphosphatemia
Hypophosphatemia	Low levels of phosphorus in the blood	No symptoms unless levels are critically low and then respiratory problems, irritability, confusion or coma can occur	Treating the underlying condition, magnesium or vitamin D supplements	At risk for respiratory compromise r/t hypophosphatemia
Potassium 3.7 to 5.2 mEq/L				
Hyperkalemia	High levels of potassium in the blood	Nausea, muscle fatigue, arrhythmias, paralysis, and weakness.	Treating the underlying cause In some cases Kexelate is needed to eliminate excessive potassium	At risk for cardiac dysfunction r/t hyperkalemia
Hypokalemia	Low levels of potassium in the blood	Dysrhythmias, constipation, palpitations, fatigue, muscle weakness, spasms, tingling or numbness	Potassium replacement and a diet rich in potassium	Muscular weakness r/t hypokalemia

Sodium 135 to 145 mEq/L				
Hypernatremia	High levels of sodium in the blood	Agitation, thirst, restlessness, coma and convulsions	Managing the underlying cause. Reducing the sodium level too quickly can cause cerebral edema, convulsions and permanent brain damage, therefore it is crucial that the client be monitored closely	At risk for convulsion and coma r/t hypernatremia
Hyponatremia	Low levels of sodium in the blood	Confusion, nausea, headache, vomiting, seizures, muscle weakness, spasms, cramps, fatigue, restlessness and irritability	Identification and management of the underlying cause, intravenous sodium and hormone replacement if Addison's disease is the cause.	Altered levels of cognition r/t hyponatremia

<u>Fatigue</u>

Fatigue is defined as extreme tiredness, a state of continuous exhaustion and a decreased ability to do physical and mental work at one's normal level of activity. Fatigue can be caused by a number of physical and psychological causes. For example, terminal disease and generalized weakness lead to fatigue; and depression, anxiety and stressful life events, like terminal disease, can lead to fatigue.

Signs and Symptoms

Some of the signs and symptoms of fatigue include decreased concentration, drowsiness, inability to perform one's usual activities, decreased libido, lack of motivation, lethargy, listlessness and guilt about not being able to fulfill one's responsibilities.

Treatment

A complete assessment is done to determine the cause of the fatigue. The level of fatigue can be assessed on a 0 to 10 scale, like pain assessment, with 0 indicating no fatigue, 1 is minimal fatigue and 10 is the greatest possible level of fatigue. It can also be quantitatively assessed according to the number of fatigue events each week including the time of day and also using a standardized fatigue scale like the Profile of Mood State Short Form Fatigue Subscale, the Multidimensional Assessment of Fatigue or the Lee Fatigue Scale, the Multidimensional Fatigue Inventory, the HIV Related Fatigue Scale, the Brief Fatigue Inventory and the Dutch Fatigue Scale.

Interventions are based on the level of fatigue and the cause of the fatigue. Some alternative treatment options include nutritional support, sleep promotion measures, the correction of biological causes, such as anemia and the effects of some medications, and psychosocial support.

Related Nursing Diagnoses

- Disturbed energy and/or motivational level r/t fatigue
- Impaired participation in care r/t fatigue
- Altered role function r/t fatigue

Diabetes

Type 1 Diabetes

Type 1 diabetes is a condition in which the insulin producing beta cells of the pancreas are attacked and destroyed by the immune system. It has autoimmune origins, because there are anti-insulin and anti-islet cell antibodies present in the blood. This pathophysiological autoimmune effect leads to lymphocytic infiltration and the destruction of the pancreas' islets. This type of diabetes will not respond to insulin-stimulating oral drugs, it requires insulin therapy by IV or injection.

It is a rapid onset disease that can occur over a few days to a week in time. Other autoimmune conditions related to Type 1 diabetes are hypothyroidism and vitiligo, which is a skin condition that is characterized by patchy depigmentation of skin on the extremities, such as the hands.

MODY

Maturity-onset diabetes of the young, or MODY, is associated with the mutation of the gene that encodes a protein called glucokinase. Insulin production fails without normal glucokinase.

Type 2 Diabetes

Type 2 diabetes results from a relative deficiency of insulin; obesity, the main cause of type 2 diabetes, causes deficiency in beta cells and peripheral insulin resistance. Patients will, over time, need to take insulin as eventually oral drugs will no longer be able to stimulate insulin release.

Gestational Diabetes

When a pregnant woman has excessive counter-insulin hormones of pregnancy it causes gestational diabetes. This results in high blood sugar and a state of insulin resistance in the pregnant woman. There may also be defective insulin receptors.

Acute Complications of Diabetes

Diabetes can lead to both acute and chronic complications. All of these complications can be prevented with the close monitoring of blood glucose levels, medications, diet and exercise.

Some of the acute complications of diabetes include hypoglycemia, hyperglycemia, diabetic ketoacidosis (DKA) and hyperglycemic hyperosmolar nonketotic syndrome (HHNS.) All diabetic clients should be fully knowledgeable about the signs, symptoms, prevention and treatment of all of these acute complications of diabetes.

Hypoglycemia

Hypoglycemia, or low blood glucose, is defined as a blood glucose level that is less than 70 mg/dL. Some of the early warning signs and symptoms of diabetic hypoglycemia include dizziness, headache, slurred speech, sweating, anxiety, shakiness, irritability and hunger. Late, and more severe symptoms, include double vision, convulsions and seizures, unconsciousness, confusion, agitation, slurred speech and clumsiness. Severe hypoglycemia leads to coma and death.

Hypoglycemia can generally be treated by the oral ingestion of glucose tablets or sugar, which can consist of candy or fruit juice. An injection of glucagon or intravenous glucose can be administered if the client is unable to orally ingest sugar

Related Nursing Diagnoses

- At risk for convulsion r/t hypoglycemia
- At risk for coma and death r/t hypoglycemia

Hyperglycemia

Hyperglycemia, or high blood glucose, is defined as a fasting (8hour) blood glucose level that is more than 180 mg/dL. Despite the fact that hyperglycemia leads to complications and chronic diabetes disorders, it, unlike hypoglycemia is not life threatening.

Hyperglycemia symptoms do not occur until the client's blood glucose level exceeds 200 mg/dL.

The early signs and symptoms include headache, fatigue, blurred vision, excessive thirst and frequent urination. If these early symptoms are left untreated, ketones, or toxic acids, will build up in the client's blood and urine (ketoacidosis.)

If hyperglycemia is left untreated there are several long-term complications that can result. These chronic, long term complications are fully discussed below.

A client can keep their blood glucose levels within a normal range by exercising regularly, taking their medications as directed, and adjusting their insulin doses as needed to prevent hyperglycemia.

Related Nursing Diagnoses

- At risk for long term complications of diabetes r/t hyperglycemia
- Knowledge deficit r/t blood glucose control

Diabetic Ketoacidosis

Signs and Symptoms

The signs and symptoms of diabetic ketoacidosis usually develop quickly, often within 24 hours, and they include nausea and vomiting, abdominal pain, weakness or fatigue, shortness of breath, fruity-scented breath, confusion, excessive thirst, and frequent urination.

Diabetic ketoacidosis is treated with a three step process of:

- Rehydration, which includes oral or intravenous fluids to dilute the excess sugar in the client's urine and to replace fluids that have been lost from excessive urination

- Intravenous electrolytes to prevent any short and long term complications that can adversely affect the client's heart, muscles and nervous system

- Intravenous insulin therapy until the client's blood sugar level falls below 240 mg/dL and is no longer acidic

Related Nursing Diagnoses

- At risk for cardiac complications r/t ketoacidosis

- Knowledge deficit r/t the signs, symptoms and prevention of ketoacidosis

Hyperglycemic Hyperosmolar Nonketotic Syndrome (HHNS)

Initial signs and symptoms of hyperglycemic hyperosmolar nonketotic syndrome (HHNS) include fever, convulsions, lethargy, nausea, weight loss, coma, confusion, weakness, increased thirst, and increased urination. If left untreated, other symptoms can develop over a period of days to weeks, including speech impairments, loss of feeling or function of one's muscles and dysfunctional movement.

The possible complications related to hyperglycemic hyperosmolar nonketotic syndrome are acute respiratory collapse or shock, blood clotting, cerebral edema, and lactic acidosis.

The treatment of hyperglycemic hyperosmolar nonketotic syndrome includes intravenous fluids with potassium, intravenous insulin and other medications to correct any problems relating to the client's blood pressure, urinary output, level of hydration and circulation.

Related Nursing Diagnoses

- At risk for acute respiratory collapse and shock r/t hyperglycemic hyperosmolar nonketotic syndrome
- Cerebral edema r/t hyperglycemic hyperosmolar nonketotic syndrome

Chronic Complications of Diabetes

Unmanaged and poorly controlled diabetes can lead to a wide variety of complications, including those that lead to severe disability and even death. A large number of these complications are related to the vascular damage that diabetes causes in terms of both the microvascular, or microcirculation, and macrovascular, or macrovascular circulation. The control of blood glucose at HbA1c < 7% can prevent these complications.

Microvascular Damage

Microvascular damage leads to many of the most commonly occurring complications of diabetes, namely, retinopathy, nephropathy and neuropathy. It can also lead to alterations of the integumentary system which places the client at risk for poor wound healing, ulcerations, and infections, particularly those affecting the lower extremities, or legs and feet.

Retinopathy

Sadly, this preventable complication of diabetes is the leading cause of adult blindness in our nation. Pathophysiologically, capillary microaneurysms occur in the retina which is followed with macular edema. Although the initial stage of diabetic retinopathy is often asymptomatic, it later leads to blurred vision, detachment of the retina or vitreous, and finally a loss of vision, which can be partial or complete. The rate of progression varies among individuals.

Nephropathy

Diabetic nephropathy, a renal glomerular disorder, includes the sclerosis of the glomeruli, a thickening of the glomerular membrane, and mesangial expansion. These pathophysiological changes lead to decreased glomerular filtration rates and glomerular hypertension.

This diagnosis is based on the presence of urinary albumin. A ratio > 30 mg/g or an albumin excretion 30 to 300 mg/24 h suggests the early stage of diabetic nephropathy. Advanced diabetic nephropathy is signaled with a positive urine dipstick for protein which indicates that the albumin excretion is more than 300 mg/day.

Treatment aims to control the client's blood pressure and the client's control of their blood glucose. An ACE inhibitor, an angiotensin II receptor blocker, or a combination of both may be indicated to control the client's hypertension.

Neuropathy

This complication of diabetes consists of nerve ischemia, or death, as the result of a combination of metabolic changes within the cells that alter nerve fiber functioning, the direct effects of high glucose levels on nerve neurons and ischemia in the microvascular circulation.

There are multiple types of diabetic neuropathy including symmetric polyneuropathy, referred to as the "stocking glove" type of neuropathy because it affects the hands and the feet, autonomic neuropathy which can affect all aspects of the autonomic nervous system and can manifest with nausea, vomiting, gastroparesis, orthostatic hypotension, tachycardia, constipation, diarrhea and dumping syndrome, urinary and fecal incontinence, diminished vaginal lubrication, erectile dysfunction and urinary retention. Other types are symmetric polyneuropathy which decreases ankle reflexes and sensory functioning, radiculopathies which lead to pain, weakness and atrophy of the lower extremities, and, finally, cranial neuropathy which can adversely affect the 3rd cranial nerve (the oculomotor nerve), the 4th cranial nerve (the trochlear nerve), and the 6th cranial nerve (the abducens nerve.)

Atherosclerosis

Large vessel, macrovascular, atherosclerosis is characterized by the possibility of myocardial infarction (MI), angina pectoris, peripheral artery disease, strokes (cerebrovascular accidents) and transient ischemic attacks (TIA.)

Cardiomyopathy

Diabetic cardiomyopathy can occur as the result of hypertension, left ventricular hypertrophy, microvascular impairments, obesity, metabolic disturbances and atherosclerosis, among other causes. Diabetic clients with cardiomyopathy are at greater risk than others for heart failure, myocardial infarction (MI) and heart failure after a myocardial infarction.

Infections

Infections of all types are an ongoing threat to the client with diabetes mellitus. The hyperglycemia of diabetes impairs the normal functioning of the T cells and granulocytes that normally protect the body from infections. Fungal infections, such as vaginal and oral candidiasis (thrush), and bacterial infections of the foot are common. Lower extremity impairments as the result of diabetic neuropathy, immunosuppression, and circulatory impairments compound the risk of foot and leg infections. Diabetic foot complications can lead to the loss of a limb when ulcerations, infections and gangrene occur.

Mononeuropathy

Mononeuropathies, another complication of diabetes, can cause foot drop, finger numbness, weakness and carpal tunnel syndrome, among other nerve compressions of the medial nerve.

Related Nursing Diagnoses

- At risk for acute and chronic complications r/t diabetes
- Risk for ineffective peripheral tissue perfusion r/t impaired circulation
- Neuropathy or nephropathy r/t uncontrolled diabetes

IMMUNE/LYMPHATIC SYMPTOMS

Infection and Fever

A fever is an important defense against infection. Almost all infections cause fevers.

Signs and Symptoms

Malaise, anorexia, depression, lethargy, hyperalgesia (an increased sensitivity to pain), and sleepiness are the most common signs of a fever in addition to the signs of local or systemic infection.

Treatment

Antipyretic medications like acetaminophen, ibuprofen and aspirin are used as well as cool compresses.

Related Nursing Diagnoses

Hyperalgesia r/t fever
Lethargy and anorexia r/t fever

Myelosupression

Myelosuppression, also referred to as bone marrow suppression or myelotoxicity, is defined as a decrease in cells that are responsible for carrying oxygen, providing immunity, and normal blood clotting. Myelosuppression is a common side effect of chemotherapy and, although it has no symptoms itself, there are many adverse conditions that can result from it.

Signs and Symptoms

Myelosuppression is a painless condition with which decreases vitally important blood cells and can result in fatigue, an increased risk of infection, excessive bleeding, and, depending on its severity, can be life-threatening.

Treatment

If the cause of myelosuppression is from chemotherapy or radiation, these treatments may have to be stopped, delayed or reduced in terms of intensity. Red blood cells can be replaced with transfusions, packed red blood cells or platelets. Other treatment options include the injection of growth factors, vitamins and antibiotics.

Related Nursing Diagnoses

At risk for infection r/t myelosuppression

At risk for hemorrhage r/t myelosuppression

Anemia

Anemia, which is very common in cancer patients and others at the end of life, is a decrease in the oxygen carrying red blood cells. There are several types of anemia including folic acid deficiency anemia, iron deficiency anemia, hemolytic anemia, sickle cell anemia and Cooley's anemia, which is also known as thalassemia. Anemia can arise from a number of causes including cancers like Hodgkin's disease and lymphoma, chronic kidney disease, infections, such as endocarditis, HIV/AIDS and hepatitis, liver cirrhosis, and some autoimmune disorders, such as systemic lupus erythematosus, and Crohn's disease.

Signs and Symptoms

The signs and symptoms include shortness of breath, dizziness, fatigue, pale skin, which normally affects the lips and nail beds, and an increased heart rate.

Treatment

Anemia is treated according to its cause and its severity. Iron supplementation, blood transfusions, and erythropoietin for clients with renal disease are some of the treatment options.

Neutropenia

Neutropenia is a decrease in the number of white blood cells, or neutrophils, in the body which serve the immune system with protection against infections. Neutropenia can be caused by leukemia, radiation therapy, chemotherapy, some medications like psychotropic medications, a nutritional deficiency, diminished bone marrow production of neutrophils, some infections, such as tuberculosis and Epstein-Barr virus, and an abnormal destruction of the neutrophils outside of the bone marrow.

Signs and Symptoms

Neutropenia can present with the signs of infection, diarrhea and rash.

Treatment

The treatment can include the elimination of medication-related causes, granulocyte colony-stimulating factor (G-CSF), which stimulates the bone marrow to produce more white blood cells, treating the infection that may have caused it, and the protection of the immunocompromised client from infections.

Thrombocytopenia

Thrombocytopenia is a drop in the number of platelets in the blood. Platelets facilitate clotting, so thrombocytopenia causes abnormal bleeding. Low platelets can occur when an insufficient amount is not produced by the bone marrow, when platelets abnormally breakdown in the blood and when platelets are destroyed by the liver or spleen.

Thrombocytopenia can occur as the result of cancers affecting the bone marrow, like leukemia, chemotherapy, myelodysplasia, a vitamin B 12 deficiency, disseminated intravascular coagulation, some medications, immune disorders, aplastic anemia, liver cirrhosis and folate deficiencies.

Signs and Symptoms

Some of the signs and symptoms are easy bruising, nosebleeds, mouth and gum bleeding, and petechiae.

Treatment

Thrombocytopenia caused b y chemotherapy will usually dissipate after the treatment is done; other treatments include platelet transfusions, bone marrow transplantation, and growth factor injections.

Lymphedema

Lymphedema is the abnormal swelling of the arm(s) and/or leg(s) that results from a blockage in the lymphatic system that normally drains the lymphatic fluid.

Signs and Symptoms

The signs and symptoms of lymphedema are restricted range of motion and swelling in the arm or leg, aching or discomfort, hardening and thickening of the skin, a feeling of heaviness and recurring infections in the affected limb.

Treatment

The treatment focuses on making the client more comfortable, which can include ice to reduce inflammation and help numb the pain. Other treatments include light exercise that can help the fluid move out of the client's limb and back into the circulatory system, wrapping the affected area in ace bandages, massage, which is known as manual lymph drainage, pneumatic compression and compression garments that apply pressure on the fluid to drain it from the affected area and other forms of decongestive therapy.

Related Nursing Diagnoses

- Pain r/t excess fluid volume secondary to lymphedema
- At risk for bleeding r/t thrombocytopenia

- At risk for infection r/t neutropenia
- Fatigue r/t decreased oxygen supply to the body (anemia)
- Ineffective protection r/t bleeding disorder

MENTAL STATUS CHANGES

Agitation and Terminal Restlessness

With time, terminally ill clients may, surprisingly to their loved ones, become agitated and restless. The degree to which they are agitated or restless can vary greatly among clients.

Terminally ill clients may experience profound mood changes when initially diagnosed, throughout the perideath progression of the disease process and/or during the final moments and hours of life. These changes are often difficult for their loved ones to handle.

Signs and Symptoms

Clients who experience this restlessness or agitation often present signs and symptoms, such as complaining of discomfort, yelling out in an uncharacteristic language, hallucinations, psychotic episodes, and loss of control. The client's safety and the safety of others can often be at risk during agitation or restlessness.

When nearing death, the terminally ill experience organ failure including poor renal and hepatic function, which accumulates retained bodily waste products, dramatic changes to the pH of the blood, and a dramatic imbalance of chemical and biological homeostasis. Severe agitation and restlessness can often occur as the result of these changes.

Treatment

When a treatable underlying cause is not identified and treated, the client may be given antianxiety medications like lorazepam and diazepam, and antipsychotic medications like haloperidol and chlorpromazine HCl.

Related Nursing Diagnoses

- Anxiety and restlessness r/t end of life changes
- At risk for physical injury r/t end of life agitation and restlessness

Confusion

Acute confusion leads to disturbances of the client's cognition, perception and attention, which can often be reversed; however, a client with chronic confusion experiences irreversible, long lasting, and/or progressive deterioration that affects their intellect and personality.

Signs and Symptoms

The signs and symptoms of acute confusion include increased agitation, lack of motivation, poor goal-directed behavior and purposeful behavior, hallucinations, cognitive fluctuations, altered levels of conscious and psychomotor activity, and increased restlessness.

The signs and symptoms of chronic confusion include impaired short-term memory, alterations in personality, altered interpretation of, and responses to, stimuli, long and short-term memory impairment, an unchanged level of consciousness, and altered intellectual abilities.

Treatment

Depending on the cause of the confusion, it can be treated. For example, confusion resulting from hypoglycemia can be treated with a piece of candy or a sweetened drink and if the confusion is a result of a fluid imbalance, the client may be given fluids and electrolytes.

Related Nursing Diagnoses

- At risk for confusion r/t end of life symptoms
- At risk for injury r/t confusion

Hallucinations

Hallucinations are sensations created by the client's mind that appear as though they are very real to them. These sensations have the ability to affect all five of the client's senses. For example, a client may see an image that no one else sees; they can hear a noise that is not heard by others; and they can smell the scent of a rose when no flowers are present.

Signs and Symptoms

Common signs and symptoms that a client can experience with hallucinations include feeling bodily sensations, such as crawling on the skin or their internal organs moving, hearing sounds, such as footsteps, banging of windows and/or doors, voices that are not truly occurring, seeing phantom lights, objects or beings, and phantom smells, such as foul or pleasant odors.

Treatment

All treatment for hallucinations depends on the underlying cause. For example if a client is experiencing hallucinations from psychosis the physician will prescribe a medication, such as dopamine antagonists.

Related Nursing Diagnoses

- At risk for injury r/t hallucinations
- Distress r/t hallucinations

IV. CARE OF THE PATIENT AND FAMILY

IDENTIFYING GOALS AND OUTCOMES

After the assessment and diagnosis stage of the nursing, the planning phase begins. Establishing patient/client goals and expected outcomes is part of the planning phase.

The SMARTTA framework can be used for setting goals or expected outcomes. All goals have to be:

- **S=** Specific
- **M=** Measurable
- **A=** Achievable
- **R=** Realistic
- **T=** Timeframe
- **T=** Trackable
- **A=** Agreed to by the client and significant other(s)

All expected outcomes must be specific and well defined and not vague. Vague goals are not useful; they are too ambiguous to direct actions. Goals must also be achievable and realistic, as based on the client's current status. For example, ambulation two times a day may not be realistic and achievable for a client who has just had a cerebrovascular accident or stroke. A more realistic and achievable goal for this client may be that the "Client will transfer from the bed to the chair with assistance two times a day."

Expected outcomes and goals must be within a timeframe that is realistic, achievable, trackable and measureable. Goals without deadlines are rarely met. The evaluation phase of the nursing process, as stated previously, is based on the measurement of preestablished goals. For this reason, goals and expected outcomes must be trackable and measurable.

The components of a well phrased expected outcome consist of a:

- *Subject*

    The subject can be the client, spouse, caregiver or significant other, but under no circumstances should it be the nurse.

    For example, it should start with the "The client will...", "The caregiver will...", or the "The spouse will..."

- *Verb*

    The verb is an action word that the subject will do, demonstrate or verbalize.

For example, the verb can be "ambulate", "list" or "will be." The goal will begin with, "the client will be able to demonstrate wound dressing changes…" or the "caregiver will list the food groups…" or the "spouse will demonstrate the procedure for taking blood glucose…"

- *Conditions*

    Conditions describe the when, how, and where of the action word or verb. For example, a condition may be "twice a day" or "with help."

- *Performance Criteria*

    Performance criteria describe exactly what is expected. It can precisely state what is expected in terms of accuracy, frequency, or time.

    For example, a performance criterion like 20 feet and twice a day can be inserted into an expected outcome, or client goal, like "The client will ambulate 20 feet with assistance two times per day." In this goal, 20 feet is the performance criteria; the subject is "client"; the verb is "ambulate"; and the condition is "with assistance."

    The best way to author expected outcomes is to state, "The client will…" or the "The wife will…" and then follow this statement with what exactly you can expect the patient or spouse to do. For example, "The client will ambulate at least 20 feet three times a day with a walker" is a good expected outcome. It is client centered ("The client will"), specific in terms of exactly what you expect the client to do, measurable in terms of feet and frequency, in a timeframe, trackable, and presumably realistic and agreed to and understood by the client (the patient, spouse, caregiver, etc..)

    Collaboration and the active involvement of the client, and significant others, must be in agreement with and must also fully understand all the client goals, or expected outcomes.

DEVELOPING A PLAN AND EVALUATING PROGRESS

The planning phase of the nursing process should be dynamic and ever changing, as based on the needs of the client and the environment. However, for the purpose of this discussion, there are three basic categories of planning in the healthcare environment:

- *Initial planning*

    Initial planning is done upon initial client contact. This initial client contact can occur when a client is admitted into an acute care facility like a hospital or medical center; it can be done upon entry into school or a prison; it can be done when a resident enters a nursing home or assisted living facility; it can be done when the client is admitted to the emergency department of an acute care facility and it can be done when a client is admitted into home care, hospice care, respite care, and an outpatient drug rehabilitation facility.

    This initial planning should be completed as soon as possible after the first client contact in order to ensure that the client will receive timely and appropriate care.

- *Ongoing planning*

    Ongoing planning, which is often neglected, is planning done in a continuous, ongoing manner in order to ensure that the plan of care accurately and completely reflects the current, ever changing client condition and changing priorities of care.

    Failures to perform ongoing planning can lead to the lack of timely and appropriate care that is based on the client's current condition. When the client's condition is changing in a rapid manner, such as minute to minute, the plan of care must be done minute by minute.

- *Discharge planning*

    Like initial planning, discharge planning should, and must, commence at the time of the first client contact. Discharge planning typically reflects the ongoing care of the client along the continuum of care. For example, a discharge plan may include home health care, hospice and palliative care, or nursing home considerations.

    Failures to plan discharges along the continuum of care are costly and very preventable when ongoing assessments/planning is complete and accurate.

Evaluating Progress Toward Expected Outcomes and Updating Goals

Evaluation consists of comparing data related to the client's current condition to the preestablished expected outcomes of care that were established during the planning phase of the nursing process. Were the goals completely met? Were the goals only partially met?

Were the goals not met at all? After these determinations, the nurse decides to continue, modify, or discontinue part of the plan of care.

The five steps of the evaluation process are:

1. Data collection relating to the expected outcome
2. Data analysis and comparison of the data to the outcomes
3. Relating the interventions to the expected outcomes
4. Concluding about the client's problem status
5. Making a decision about whether to continue the plan of care, or to modify it or to discontinue it

After the evaluation is complete, the nurse will generate and document an evaluation statement that begins with one of these three alternatives:

- Goal was met
- Goal was partially met
- Goal was not met

When the goals are met, the goals are discontinued; when a goal was partially met, the nurse may change it or leave it as it is and continue with the planned interventions. Lastly, when there is no movement toward the goal, the entire nursing process, starting with assessment, is done again to identify any areas that are missing and/or not accurate.

RESOURCE MANAGEMENT

Medicare and Medicaid

The United State's Medicare administered program and the state-level Medicaid programs are two primary governmental reimbursement programs. Medicare, under the U.S. Social Security Act, reimburses for the health care of adults who are 65 years of age and older, and some younger permanently disabled people and their dependents. Medicaid, on the other hand, provides healthcare reimbursement for low-income individuals, families and chronically ill children.

Medicare Hospice Benefits

Medicare hospice benefits include two 90-day benefit periods and an unlimited number of 60-day benefit periods as long as the client continues to meet the eligibility criteria under Medicare Part A benefits. Admission criteria include the fact that the client is deemed terminally ill with less than six months to live. The medical director of the hospice and the client's attending physician document this initial certification.

When the client elects hospice care, they sign an election form waiving their rights to all Medicare benefits, such as the treatment of the terminal condition and care over and above what was designated in the election form. For more information about hospice care reimbursement go to the below link:

http://www.cgsmedicare.com/hhh/education/materials/pdf/Medicare_Hospice_Benefit_Facts.pdf

Medicaid Hospice Benefits

All states throughout the nation, and the District of Columbia, provide Medicaid coverage for hospice care, with the exception of the state of Oklahoma. Oklahoma provides hospice care reimbursement only to those with the Advantage Waiver. Additionally, Medicaid does not provide reimbursement for hospice care in any of its territories, like Guam and American Samoa.

The criteria, coverage limitations and reimbursement methodologies vary among states so it is recommended that you research your state's Medicaid regulations relating to hospice care. However, all states are required to provide the same four levels of care as Medicare, as was discussed above.

Third Party Private Insurance Companies

Most, if not all, third party private insurance companies reimburse for hospice care. The benefits, admission criteria, coverage limitations and reimbursement methods, however, may vary somewhat so if you are managing reimbursements for your clients, check with the individual's specific insurance company for their specific requirements and benefits.

Providing Education about Access to Services, Medications, Supplies and Durable Medical Equipment

Medicare Part A, as stated, covers hospital, skilled nursing, and hospice care. Part B medical insurance includes physician and nursing services, renal dialysis, laboratory and other diagnostic tests, blood transfusions, chemotherapy, immunosuppressive drugs for organ transplant clients, prosthetic devices, oxygen, and durable medical equipment like canes, walkers, and wheelchairs.

Clients and family members should be educated and informed about Medicare, Medicaid and how to access necessary supplies, services and durable medical equipment.

Accommodating Socioeconomic Factors

Nurses, and other members of the healthcare team, including case managers and social workers, assess the client's socioeconomic status upon admission and determine if there are any socioeconomic issues that need to be addressed.

ASSESSING SAFETY AND RESPONDING TO ENVIRONMENTAL RISKS

Falls and Falls Prevention

Falls are one of the biggest, and most costly, patient-related accidents in health care. All clients should be screened and assessed for falls risk upon admission. If the client has been identified as at risk for falls, special interventions and preventive measures must be immediately implemented.

Some of the risk factors associated with falls include:

- *Poor vision*

    People who are visually impaired are at risk for tripping over objects difficult to see, particularly in a strange or new environment. Clients should be given their eyeglasses and encouraged to use them.

- *Slow reaction time*

    Older people to react to dangers more slowly than younger people. For example, an elderly person may be unable to react quickly enough to avoid a hazard on the floor and fall as a result.

- *Incontinence*

    Patients who are incontinent of feces and/or urine are at greater risk for falls than clients who are not affected with these elimination problems.

- *Confusion*

    People who are confused may lack good judgment and they may not be aware of any hazards.

- *Environmental hazards*

    Environmental areas that have clutter, poor light, high glare, and wet floors are not safe. The nurse, and all members of the team, are responsible to keep the client environment safe and without any hazards.

- *Age*

    Older people fall more than young people. Infants and young children are also at risk for falls. Infants, young children and elderly adults are most at risk for injuries and accidents.

- *Medications*

    Sedation, other medications and medication side effects, such as orthostatic hypotension, place clients at risk for falls.

- *Poor balance, coordination, gait and range of motion (ROM)*

    When unable to safely maintain balance, an individual will fall. It is not unusual for patients to demonstrate a poor gait and poor balance, resulting in lack of coordination and diminished muscular range of motion. The assistance of a physical therapist may be highly beneficial to these clients.

- *Past falls*

    Those patients and residents with a history of falling risk future falls, while patients who have fallen more than once are at a particularly high risk of falling again.

- *Fear of falling*

    Patients afraid of falling will stiffen, tensing and tightening their muscles; these physical manifestations of fear of falling may, in fact, lead to a fall.

- *Weak muscles*

    People who have muscular weakness, paralysis and/or neuropathy require help and care to avoid falls.

- *Some diseases and disorders*

    A client who has a seizure disorder, arthritis, a stroke or Parkinson's disease is, for example, at risk for falls.

- *Patient footwear*

    Patients require skid-proof shoes or slippers that fit; otherwise, footwear itself is a hazard.

- *Broken equipment*

    Broken equipment like canes, walkers, wheelchairs or wheelchair brakes are hazardous, can lead to falls, and should NEVER be used. Report ALL broken equipment and remove it from service immediately.

Preventing falls is a team effort. Take special measures immediately for any patient or resident at assessed at being at risk for falls to ensure proper nursing care.

Biological Safety: Infection Control and Nosocomial Infections

Most nosocomial infections are spread by the hands of health care workers from one patient to another. These infections are limited to only those infections that a patient did not have before they were hospitalized, or cared for, but acquired after admission or after care was provided.

The most commonly occurring risk factors for nosocomial infections are prolonged illness and immunosuppression, treatments such as chemotherapy, invasive procedures, like indwelling urinary catheters, and some medications. Additionally, all pieces of equipment and nonsterile supplies can harbor and spread nosocomial infections. Nosocomial infections are very costly and they can, for the most part, be prevented.

The urinary tract, the respiratory tract, wounds, and the bloodstream are the most common sites for nosocomial infections; and some of the commonly occurring pathogens include E. coli, Candida albicans, staphylococcus aureus, pseudomonas aeruginosa, and enterococcus.

Hand washing is the single most effective way to prevent nosocomial infections in our healthcare facilities. Protective precautions, such as standard precautions and transmission-based precautions, are also necessary, particularly because of the presence of so many resistant strains of pathogens, like methicillin-resistant staphylococcus aureus (MRSA), vancomycin resistant enterococcus (VRE) and penicillin resistant streptococcus pneumoniae.

Protective precautions include:

- Standard precautions that apply to all blood and bodily fluids and all clients regardless of the person's diagnosis

- Contact precautions to prevent any direct and indirect contact transmissions, as those contained in diarrhea, wounds, and herpes simplex.

- Airborne precautions for the prevention of airborne transmission microbes like TB. These precautions include a HEPA mask and a negative pressure room.

- Droplet precautions are used to prevent the transmission of pathogens that are transmitted with a cough or sneeze. Masks are indicated for these precautions.

Oxygen Therapy Safety

There are a number of precautions that need to be taken to allow for safety with oxygen therapy.

These safety precautions include educating the client, family and visitors about the dangers of smoking and open flames, the placement of a no smoking sign in the home, avoiding static electricity by using only cotton fiber linens, blankets and clothing around oxygen therapy, avoiding the use of electric devices, such as electric razors and hairdryers, anywhere near oxygen therapy, insuring that the electrical medical equipment is grounded, keeping flammable materials, such as nail polish, alcohol or acetone, away from oxygen therapy, and placing and knowing the location of the nearest fire extinguisher.

Adapting the Patient's Environment for Safety

Nurses and other members of the healthcare team must ensure client safety. At times, the services of a physical therapist may be indicated; and at other times modifications of the environment and assistive devices are needed.

Modifications of the Environment

Safe rooms and patient care areas are well lit and void of hazards. There should be no cords, wires, clutter, or other potential tripping hazards present. Rooms should be clean and dry, without skidding or slipping risks. Rooms should have grab bars and handrails for patients, particularly in bathrooms and in areas where they walk. Chairs should be stable and equipped with armrests. Patient independence must be balanced with patient safety; thus, frequent monitoring is necessary.

Assistive Devices

The primary purposes of assistive devices for mobility are to enhance the client's ability to overcome environmental barriers, to lessen the impact of a temporary or permanent functional locomotive impairment, to maintain balance, stability, and strength, as well as to increase and maintain the client's independent function, despite a disability.

All assistive and adaptive devices must be in proper and safe condition and they must also be fitted according to the client's specific characteristics and needs.

Transfer Training and Exercises

Transfers are essential for all out of bed activities. Patients have a need to exit the bed and transfer to a chair or another device like a stretcher. They also have to be able to transfer from a toilet, commode, wheelchair, shower, bathtub, and/or automobile. Safe transfers require balance, muscular strength, joint mobility and physical stamina. Some clients who have the rehabilitation potential for safe transfers need the collaborative assistance of the physical therapist and nurses to regain, restore or improve their transfer abilities.

Other clients with no potential for safe transfers need alternative mechanical devices such as a hydraulic lift or complete assistance with transfers by lifting the client using proper body mechanics, sturdy lift sheets, lifting boards, and the help of several nurses. Lastly, there are clients who can assist with transfers so the nurse or another member of the team, will then assist the client with a pivot transfer, provided that the client can weight bear.

Monitoring Controlled Substances

Controlled substances must be securely stored in a double-locked cabinet; when using them, their removal must be immediately recorded and documented on the narcotic record. This documentation is NOT done after the medication is administered; it is documented immediately upon removal from a secured location.

Immediately after administering them, narcotics are documented in the patient's medication record. If a controlled substance is partially or entirely unused (wasted), this waste must be witnessed by the wasting nurse and another nurse. Two nurses document this wasting.

Opioid use, misuse and diversion are a major concern in healthcare and in society. Prescription drug use and misuse is the most frequent form of drug abuse in the community and, sadly, some healthcare professionals, like doctors and nurses, may also use, misuse and divert medications from clients.

The diversion of controlled substances leads to several adverse outcomes including risks to the person who is diverting the drugs, risks to clients and their safety, and risks in terms of employer vulnerability.

Preventive measures should be failsafe and effective. Multiple departments in the healthcare facility should be actively engaged in preventive measures along the entire process of medication administration, from ordering to documentation. Nursing, pharmacy, security, anesthesiology, legal counsel, administration, and human resources departments, as well as others, must be involved and actively engaged. Policies and procedures and reporting systems must be complete, thorough and effective.

Identifying Available Community Resources

It is necessary that the nurse collaborate with the client and significant others to identify all of the available community resources that may be of benefit to them. Some of these community resources can include social support and counseling agencies, community service agencies, volunteers, home care nursing agencies, and peer support groups or self-help groups.

PSYCHOSOCIAL, SPIRITUAL AND CULTURAL ISSUES

Assessing and Responding to Needs

As discussed above, the client and significant others are affected with psychological, spiritual and culture needs, and these needs are assessed during the assessment phase of the nursing process and addressed in the planning and implementation phases of the nursing process.

Some of the most commonly occurring psychosocial needs for palliative care and hospice clients include anger, anxiety, denial, depression, fear, grief, guilt, loss of hope or meaning, nearing death awareness, sleep disturbances, social withdrawal and intimacy/relationship issues.

The nurse and other members of the healthcare team, including psychologists and clergy members, are often helpful in assisting the client to resolve these unresolved matters.

Assessing and Responding to Family Systems and Dynamics

Some of the most commonly occurring family dynamics issues for palliative care and hospice clients include the interrelationships of factors like family strife, interpersonal conflicts, role disintegration, geographic distance, and patterns of coping and expressing grief.

Identifying Unresolved Interpersonal Matters

Many clients at the end of life have unresolved interpersonal matters that they would like to attend to. Some of the most commonly occurring unresolved matters include making amends, apologizing for one's failures, and expressing thoughts of love and acceptance of others who the client may have not done so with in the past. Many of these end of life discussions relieve guilt and anxiety.

Again, the nurse and other members of the healthcare team, including psychologists and clergy members, are often helpful in assisting the client to resolve these unresolved matters.

Facilitating Effective Communication

Some of the factors that can affect the communication process include:

- Cultural values and beliefs
- Perception
- Attitudes
- Differences in knowledge
- Past experiences
- Emotions
- Relationships and roles

- Environmental settings
- Physical discomfort
- Time pressures

The nurse must establish and maintain therapeutic, open and nonjudgmental relationships with clients that are culturally sensitive and culturally competent. Cultural values or beliefs often differ between patients and nurses; different cultural beliefs, worldviews, vocabulary and terminology, as well as cultural practices affect human interactions and communication.

Perceptions and attitudes also influence how a message is interpreted. Effective and therapeutic communication can also be quite challenging when the sender and receiver differ in terms of their levels of education and knowledge. Because the vast majority of clients and significant others do not understand medical terminology, anatomy, physiology and disease processes, nurses should avoid medical jargon and communicate with patients in a manner that is fully understandable to the client and significant others.

Past experiences can also powerfully affect perceptions and interpretation of the meaning of messages. Negative past experiences with healthcare systems can lead to skepticism and a lack of trust on the part of the patient. Additionally, many emotions can influence how a person relates to others. Fear, pain, anger, and anxiety often adversely affect the nurse-client interaction and communication.

Relationships and roles directly affect the style and type of communication. For example, some cultures hold the male as the primary decision-maker and some patients withhold personal details about themselves until trust and a nonjudgmental relationship is established with the nurse.

The healthcare environment is not particularly conducive to good communication. Nurses must attempt to create an environment free of noise and distractions where there is privacy and comfort in order to facilitate optimal communication with clients and significant others.

Physical discomfort, fatigue, pain and anxiety adversely affect the communication process. Whenever possible, these factors should be minimized or eliminated to facilitate a good therapeutic relationship with the client.

The pressure of time and a nurse's sense of urgency to complete other tasks while they are communicating with patients interfere with effective communication. For example, a patient will not fully discuss their needs, feelings, fears and concerns when they perceive that the nurse is in a hurry.

Barriers to Therapeutic Communication

Barriers to therapeutic communication and conversation stoppers include changing the subject, defensiveness, false reassurances, probing, disagreeing, judgments, rejection and challenging.

People change the subject inappropriately when they are unwilling or too uncomfortable to discuss the subject at hand. It stops the conversation. For example, a client may perceive that the nurse is not interested in or concerned about their feelings or beliefs when the nurse changes the subject because of their own anxiety and discomfort.

"Don't worry, you will be just fine" is an example of false reassurance. Nurses often give false reassurances as the result of the nurse's inability to cope emotionally with the client's state of health, fears and feelings. False reassurances can lead the client to experience further anxiety and may cause the patient to feel as though the nurse does not care about them.

Defensiveness can be injected into the nurse-patient interaction when the nurse feels a need to defend themselves and/or the healthcare system for weaknesses and shortcomings. Clients who ask the nurse a question do not benefit from trite common advice; the nurse should offer the client professional information that enables the client to make an independent, patient-focused, and knowledgeable decision.

Challenging occurs when the nurse directly or indirectly asks the patient to justify and defend their personal beliefs, thoughts, and feelings. Challenging attacks the client and the validity of the patient's own thoughts and feelings.

Probing is invasive and it violates the patient's right to privacy. Testing is also not therapeutic. Testing occurs when the nurse asks a question that the client is forced to answer with a response that is beneficial to the nurse and not the client. For example, the nurse may ask, "Do you think that I am taking good care of you today?" The patient feels pressure to say "yes."

Stereotyping is a barrier to effective communication because it entails general statements that do not reflect individuality. Disagreeing as well as agreeing also blocks open, therapeutic communication. All client feelings and beliefs are valid and not right or wrong. Lastly, judgmental attitudes force the client to believe that they must agree with the nurse and change their own personal beliefs and concerns.

Encouraging a Life Review

Many clients nearing death experience a life review or life reconciliation. There are five stages of life review, which include expression, responsibility, forgiveness, acceptance, and gratitude.

During expression, the client oftentimes experiences anger as the most dominant emotion. It is important for the client to express their emotions and any intense feelings they may have, as well as releasing their anger in order to find peace.

In the responsibility stage, the client often realizes that they have had a part in all that has happened to them, and they realize that their thoughts, actions, and lives are their responsibility alone. This is often described as a freeing experience.

The forgiveness phase allows the client the ability to decide to let go of any hurt or resentment they may have to enable them to be at peace. It is oftentimes easier for the client to forgive others than for them to forgive themselves. Clients may choose the forgiveness route, while others choose to remain unforgiving.

The acceptance phase allows the client to accept their death as inevitable and discontinues a losing battle, which does not mean that they are not giving up on life; they are just able to accept the natural order of life that includes death. With acceptance, clients are able to experience peace and contentment in their time left.

During the gratitude phase, clients are able to experience gratitude in extreme levels for experiences they have throughout their lives, whether good or bad. They are thankful for the people who are a part of their lives, and for a God or higher power if they believe in one.

Counseling and Providing Support for Grieving Adults

Grief and loss affects different people in different ways. Emotional support is provided with individual and/or group approaches, formal and informal interventions, and by a number of healthcare professionals including nurses, social workers, psychologists, and members of the clergy.

It can be very comforting and reassuring to receive support from others when a person is affected with the effects of grief and loss. Group counseling and support can be a way for clients and significant others to share their feelings, their story and experiences. Clients can also develop supportive relationships and share information and resources. Individual counseling is also done, however, when the client has needs that are best addressed and resolved with one-to-one psychological support.

Counseling and Providing Support for Grieving Children

Children can be profoundly affected by the loss of a family member, friend, peer, and even a pet. Children may have many questions regarding the death and death process and these questions should be answered honestly.

Death, the meaning of death and the finality of death are concepts that children develop in a rather predictable manner as they mature. These beliefs and perceptions are, as follows:

- Before the age of 3 years of age: This child does not comprehend death and its permanent nature. These children do fear separation, however, and they have separation anxiety when they are not with parents and other loved ones.

- Between 3 and 5 years of age: This age group views death as reversible and they often perceive that the dead person is simply sleeping.

- Between the ages of 6 and 10: The child begins to understand the finality of death. They engage in mystical thinking that aims to avoid their own death and the death of loved ones.

- At about 11 to 12 years of age: The child fully recognizes the irreversible permanent nature of death and they begin to become interested in the afterlife.

Some interventions that facilitate the resolution of a child's grief and loss include art therapy, play therapy, age-appropriate support groups, workshops that are specialized for the child's level of development and individual counseling depending on the child and their needs.

Providing Support for a Death Vigil

Death vigils vary among individuals, families, religions, cultures and ethnic groups. Individuals vary in terms of their physical and emotional attributes and strengths. Some can, and choose to, stay near the loved one at the end of life, and others are unable to. Some families prefer that only the nuclear family, rather than the extended family, stay close and support the loved one during their final hours and moments. Some religious practices include the presence of a clergy person to perform religious practices, such as the Catholic Sacrament of the Sick. Some cultures are welcoming of all loved ones and some also have cultural practices and rituals at the end of life. Lastly, some ethnic groups have their own beliefs and practices at the end of life including those relating to the death vigil.

Nurses are also a highly important part of the death vigil. They remain in presence, or readily available, to care for and support the dying client and their loved ones. Simple measures such as providing privacy, a comfortable chair, coffee and meals are highly welcomed by family members. They also need the ongoing psychological and emotional support of the nurse at the end of life.

Providing Comfort and Dignity at Time of Death

Some essential comfort and dignity measures that should be implemented include the provision of comfort and privacy to loved ones and significant others, as well as providing the client with interventions. Ensure clean, dry skin, clean bed linens, good oral hygiene and hydration with ice chips if possible, proper turning and positioning, the management of incontinence, and the continuation of assessments and interventions relating to comfort measures like massage, pain management medications and treatment of any end of life symptoms.

7. PRONOUNCEMENT, NOTIFICATION AND TRANSPORTATION

The hospice or palliative care nurse, who is in the home or otherwise at the bedside when death occurs, supports the family and loved ones, documents the time of death and, in some cases, pronounces the client dead. Some, but not all states, allow the nurse to pronounce death, so it is necessary to check with your state practice acts and laws to determine if pronouncement is within the scope of the nurse's practice. If it is not, the nurse will contact the client's physician and other authorities, as required.

After pronouncement, the client is then transported to the morgue or funeral home according to the planned final arrangements. If an autopsy is to be performed, the body should remain undisturbed and things like tubes, lines and catheters should not be removed. If, however, an autopsy will not be done, postmortem care is done by the nurse.

Facilitating Transition to Bereavement Services

The family members and/or loved ones of the client, after death has occurred, are encouraged to acknowledge the pain of loss. The support and presence of the nurse allows the bereaved to express their feelings and to resolve their grief.

It is important that the bereaved not use any medications to suppress the pain of grieving. The nurse can support the family members and/or loved ones to grieve in a healthy, rather than a dysfunctional, manner. The acceptance of loss is the beginning phase of the healthy grieving process. Dysfunctional grieving is defined as an extended and unsuccessful resolution of grief.

The nurse can facilitate healthy grieving by encouraging the loved ones to view, touch, hold and kiss the body of their loved one and to provide emotional support at the time of death and for a period of time after the death.

Participating in Formal Closure Procedures

Nurses often become close to clients and their loved ones when they are caring for them, particularly when the nurse-client-significant relationship forms and is maintained during the perideath period.

Participating in the formal closure activities, such as visiting, calling or sending a card to the bereaved can be helpful to the bereaved as well as the nurse who cared for the client and their loved ones.

V. EDUCATION AND ADVOCACY

CAREGIVER SUPPORT

Monitoring Caregiver Confidence

Caregiver confidence and competence is a primary concern for hospice and palliative care nurses. Caregivers play a highly important role in the physical, psychological and social support of the client. Caregiver support allows the client, in many cases, to remain in their own home surrounded by loved ones and also gives the client a greater degree of comfort, self esteem, and decision-making than could occur in an environment outside of the home.

Caregivers need the support of the nurse to overcome their fears about caregiving, to learn about the client's care, to develop competency in terms of the provision of care and to develop a sense of satisfaction and confidence in terms of this role.

Education and psychosocial support facilitate caregiver confidence and the ability to provide care.

Promoting Family Self-Care Activities

The ability of the client, and the caregiver, to perform functional self-care activities is impacted by a number of factors including the individual's motivation, beliefs, needs, the environment, the cultural and ethnical background, the person's physical, psychological/emotional, spiritual wellbeing and social support. For example, the client and/or the caregiver may have barriers to self-care including fear, decreased levels of motivation, poor coping skills, musculoskeletal disabilities, nervous system impairments, poor socioeconomic status, impaired levels of cognition, and an unsafe environment.

Dorothea Orem's Self-Care theory is a good framework for nurses to use in terms of self-care by both the client and the caregiver. This theory is based on the premise that clients can, and want to, care for themselves as much as possible. The three types of nursing systems that Orem identifies are the supportive-educative (developmental), partly compensatory, and the wholly compensatory nursing systems.

The supportive-educative (developmental) nursing system aims to provide clients with the support, assistance and care that they need to continue their independent self-care. The caregiver is at this level when they are able to provide complete care to the client with only the support and education of the palliative and hospice care nurse.

The partly compensatory nursing system meets the self-care needs of those clients who can perform some, but not all self-care functions. For example, a conscious cancer client can usually perform some, but maybe not all, of their self-care activities. When the client is not able to perform some aspects of care, the caregiver should be given the knowledge, skills and abilities to help the client, and to encourage the client to perform all of the self-care skills that they can perform. The client's provision of their own self-care enhances self-esteem and self-worth. The client should be assisted only in areas of need so independence can be fostered.

Lastly, the wholly compensatory nursing system provides all care to the client because the client is not able to perform any self-care. Infants, very young children and clients in a coma are examples of clients who need wholly compensatory nursing care. At this level, it is the nurse, in collaboration with the caregiver, who provides all care to the client.

Many self-care needs include the activities of daily living (ADLs), such as personal care and hygiene, dressing, bathing, toileting, eating and drinking. One of the most important aspects of self-care is the achievement of the client's goals in terms of adaptation and independence.

Evaluating Caregiver Fatigue and Burden

Hospice and palliative care nurses must assess and evaluate the caregiver's fatigue and degree stress. Care of a loved one is often stressful and overwhelming. Caregivers need the support of the nurse. Respite care, as discussed above, and other methods of social support can be helpful, as well as other interventions which are based on the caregiver's needs.

EDUCATION

Assessing the Learner's Knowledge Base and Learning Needs

The phases of the teaching/learning process are the same as the phases of the nursing process- assessment, diagnosis, planning, implementation and evaluation.

The Assessment of Learning Needs

The purpose of assessment is to determine the client's learning needs, their level of motivation and readiness, personal, ethnical and cultural aspects, learning styles and preferences, age specific characteristics and needs, barriers to learning, including cognitive impairments, language, level of comprehension or reading level and physical as well as psychological barriers to learning. Simply stated, a learning need is what should be known minus what is actually known.

The Client/Significant Other's Knowledge Base or Entry Level Knowledge and Skills and Learning Styles

Simply stated, entry level knowledge and skills is defined as baseline knowledge and skills. The nurse assesses and determines the client's entry level knowledge and skills in order to plan appropriate educational activities to meet the client's educational needs.

Entry-level knowledge and skills consist of what the client knows at the current time and what the client can do at the current time, respectively. After this determination, the nurse compares this entry-level knowledge and skill set to what the client should know and what they should be able to do. This comparison is used to determine specific learning needs for the client.

The learning need = What the client should know – what the client actually knows now (entry level)

The learning need = What the client should be able to do – what the client can actually do now (entry level)

The assessment of entry-level knowledge and skills also gives the nurse the opportunity to identify any false knowledge, misinformation and poor self-management skills. Again, the nurse can address these deficits with planned educational activities.

Learning Styles and Preferences

People have unique learning styles and learning preferences that can facilitate or impede learning. For example, auditory learners prefer and do well with patient education discussions, but visual learners do not get the same benefits from discussions – they prefer visual information using pictures and diagrams.

Some of the learning styles and preferences include:

- Active and reflective learners
- Sensing and intuitive learners
- Verbal, auditory and tactile learners
- Sequential and global learners

All of these learning styles differ in terms of the learners' strengths and weakness and in terms of their preferred form of learning. Most people, however, have a mix, or combination, of more than one learning style. For example, a reflective learner can also have the characteristics of a verbal and/or sequential learner.

Active and Reflective Learners

Active learners prefer to learn with active engagement, doing, discussions, and group projects. Lectures without physical activity are more difficult for active learners when compared to reflective learners. Tips for Active Learners: Use group discussion and study groups.

Reflective learners prefer to learn by thinking about the learning and content material first. They prefer solitary work rather than group work. Tips for Reflective Learners: Encourage the learner to reflect on readings, contemplate applications and summarize material rather than the memorization of facts.

Sensing and Intuitive Learners

Sensing learners prefer memorizing facts, detail-oriented learning and practical, real world-oriented learning rather than abstraction. They use reliable methods of problem solving and they do not expect unanticipated results. Tips for Sensing Learners: Seek out procedures and concepts that can transform abstract concepts in concrete and practical solutions.

Intuitive learners consider relationships among various pieces of information. They prefer novel and innovative ideas rather than learning by routine. They are tolerant and welcoming of abstractions, including mathematics, and learn at a more rapid pace than sensors. Tips for Intuitive Learners: Encourage the learner to employ careful thought before answering a question and solving a problem. Encourage the learner to connect theoretical and abstract thinking to facts.

Visual, Verbal and Tactile Learners

Visual learners prefer, and learn best, when they see things. These learners benefit from flow charts, demonstrations, diagrams, medical models, and videos. Discussions are not the strategy of choice for visual learners. They benefit greatly from pictorial handouts and other visual strategies.

Verbal learners, on the other hand, benefit from the spoken and written word. Discussions and lectures are preferred over demonstration and the use of pictures.

Tactile learners tend to remember things by doing, rather than listening or reading. This type of learner tends to learn best from hands on experimentation. This type of learner tends to excel in areas such as dance, athletics or other mobility or movement based activities. Tactile learners learn through imitation and practice. There is a tendency to have difficulties with reading and comprehension.

Sequential and Global Learners

Sequential learners learn best when the material is presented with logical, orderly and linear steps; global learners, on the other hand, move the content and material all around in a seemingly illogical and disorder manner until the learner makes connections among the pieces of information and then understands it.

Sequential learners follow logical steps to find a solution and to master the material. They are also able to explain how they solved a problem. Global learners have difficulty explaining why and how the problem was solved but, nonetheless, global learners tend to have the ability to rapidly solve complex problems.

Whenever possible, the educator should employ strategies that meet the individual learning style preferences and, when, group learning is being used, the educator should employ a multitude of strategies to meet the needs and preferences of those in the group.

Identifying and Responding to Learning Barriers

Some of the barriers to learning and methods of overcoming these barriers are discussed below.

- *Literacy*

    Sadly, many people in our nation are not able to read at all. Some may only be able to read and comprehend material at a low-grade level. It is sometimes recommended that patient education material be authored at or below 6th grade reading level to accommodate for these comprehension and literacy needs.

    The nurse must assess the client's literacy level and provide learning materials that are appropriate to the client in terms of their reading level so that the person is able to benefit from them.

- *Health Literacy*

Patients are considered "health literate" when they are able to understand information and use it to make appropriate health care decisions. Almost 50% of patients are NOT health literate.

Nurses, and other healthcare professionals, must modify their communication and teaching to accommodate for this weakness and to ensure comprehension. For example, simple anatomy and physiology information relating to diabetes is preferred over complex, biochemical explanations that the client cannot understand. Additionally, the use of medical jargon and terminology should be avoided.

- *Motivation and Readiness*

Clients will not learn unless they are motivated and ready to do so. Nurses can motivate learners by involving them in the entire teaching/learning process, by focusing the learning on solving immediate and pressing concerns, by explaining the benefits of learning in terms of problem resolution, while maintaining an environment that is supportive of an open, honest and highly respectful learning environment.

Motivation to learn and motivation to change are assessed as part of the assessment phase of the teaching process. Motivation will be further discussed below.

- *Cultural Aspects*

Communication patterns, vocabulary, slang and/or terminology, are differences that separate the members of the group, or culture, from those who are not members. Nurses must become culturally competent about the cultures, norms and gestures of others, and modify our terminology and behavior according to what is acceptable and understandable to the learner.

- *Age Specific Characteristics*

Some examples of teaching modifications based on age are simple, concrete and brief explanations for the toddler, simple and brief explanations for the pre-school child, the encouragement of questions and more detailed explanations for the school-age child, and adult-like teaching for the adolescent.

- *Language Barriers*

Communicating with, and teaching, those who speak a different language can be challenging. However, these barriers can be overcome with some relatively simple techniques such as speaking slowly, clarifying, reclarifying, using pictures and diagrams, and eliciting the help of an interpreter.

- *Health Beliefs*

Health beliefs can also be a barrier to learning and changes in behavior. Clients who place a high value on health, health promotion and wellness will be more highly motivated to learn than those clients who do not place priority value on health, health promotion and wellness.

Nurses can overcome this barrier to learning by facilitating the client's understanding of the importance of these values in terms of their diabetes and ways that the person can enhance their health, health promotion and wellness, despite the presence of disease.

- *Religious and Spiritual Beliefs*

Religious and spiritual beliefs can include the use of symbols, dreams, spiritual practices and beliefs, including those that are metaphysical in nature.

For example, maintaining health may involve the use of proper clothing and proper diet (physical facet), the support of others including family members (psychological facet) and things like meditation, prayer and formalized religious practices (spiritual facet.)

Similarly, health protection is facilitated with symbolic clothing and special spiritual foods (physical facet), the avoidance of people and things that can lead to disease (psychological facet), and the use of religious customs, superstition, and amulets like the "Evil Eye" to ward off evil and harm (spiritual facet.)

Lastly, the restoration of health is enabled with alternative healing methods such as massage, herbs, homeopathic remedies and special foods (physical facet), exorcism, the use of culturally traditional healers, like medicine men and curanderos, and relaxation techniques (psychological facet) and religious rituals, special prayers, exorcism and traditional healing (spiritual facet.)

- *Family Dynamics and Other Social Forces*

Many clients have social support systems and family supports, but not all. For example, the client may be widowed, single, geographically separated from family and friends, or have no family or friends that support them and their need for education and behavior changes.

The nurse can increase social support systems by utilizing available community resources such as Meals on Wheels and transportation to and from healthcare-related services, as indicated.

- *Psychological Factors*

Nurses and other healthcare professionals have to assess and accommodate for any actual or potential cognitive, sensory and psychological/emotional barriers to learning. For example, cognitive limitations can be overcome with slow, brief, simple and understandable explanations.

Psychological barriers can be minimized with establishing trust, reinforcing learning with positive feedback, and minimizing stress. Moderate stress is a motivator; extreme stress and pain prevent learning.

- *Physical Capabilities and Limitations*

    Sensory barriers can be accommodated for with large print materials and Braille for the visually impaired, louder discussions with clients affected with a hearing loss, and the use of assistive devices like magnifiers, eyeglasses and hearing aids.

    Functional limitations can also impede learning. For example, a diabetic client who has lost fine motor coordination may not be able to draw up their own insulin without the help of some assistive devices.

Motivation and Readiness to Learn

Clients will not learn unless they are motivated and ready to do so. Nurses can motivate learners by involving them in the entire teaching/learning process, by focusing the learning on solving immediate and pressing concerns, by explain the benefits of learning in terms of problem resolution, and with the maintaining of an environment supportive of an open, honest and highly respectful learning environment. Motivation to learn and motivation to change are assessed as part of the assessment phase of the teaching process.

Some of the factors that affect motivation and readiness to learn are:

- *Level of Pain*: Clients who are in severe pain cannot learn. When at all possible, the level of pain should be decreased prior to a teaching activity.

- *Level of Stress*: Moderate levels of stress and anxiety motivate learners to learn. However, high level anxiety and stress is not conductive to learning. High stress interferes with the learner's ability to focus and concentrate on the issue at hand.

- *Developmental Level*: Some examples of teaching modifications based on age are simple concrete and brief explanations for the toddler, simple and brief explanations for the pre-school child, the encouragement of questions and more detailed explanations for the school age child, and adult like teaching for the adolescent.

- *Perceived Learning Needs*: Motivation can be affected by the client's perceptions in terms of their overall needs and the benefits that they perceive can be derived from educational activities.

- *Attitudes*: Some clients have an external locus of control and others have an internal locus of control. Clients with an external locus of control view their problems as something that occurs because of external forces and something that they have no control over. Clients with an internal locus believe that they have control.

  The locus of control can be moved from an external locus of control to an internal locus of control when the educator is able to convince the patient that they can, like so many other clients, successfully control and cope with their disease process. They develop a "can do" attitude.

Other Strategies to Enhance Motivation and Readiness

- Learning should be an extremely active and participative process.

- An explanation of the benefits of the learning to the client and family members is highly motivating because the learner believes that the teaching can help them to solve the problem.

- Relate the new knowledge to the client's past knowledge and experiences so the learner can comfortably fit this newly gained knowledge, skills and abilities into their life and life style.

- Involvement of the learners in the process of teaching and learning encourages and motivates them in learning.

- Focus on the immediate problems and concerns of the learner and family members.

- Maintain an open, honest and highly respectful learning environment.

- Encourage sharing of knowledge, ideas and past experiences with the nurse and others. Small group teaching activities provide learners with these opportunities.

Teaching Caregiver Skills

Palliative care and hospice nurses play a highly important role in caregiver education. Most caregivers enjoy, and benefit greatly from, the provision of this care to a loved one. They feel more involved and highly useful when the end of life grows near. Some of this education involves the cognitive domain of learning and other learning involves the psychomotor domain of learning. For example, caregivers learn psychomotor skills so they can provide the loved one with bathing and hygiene, and they learn about the signs and symptoms of imminent death, which is part of the cognitive domain of learning.

The Domains of Learning

There are three domains of learning that are the basis of all education, including patient and family education. These domains are the cognitive, psychomotor and affective domains.

- *The Cognitive Domain*

    This domain consists of both knowledge and understanding. An example of a cognitive domain patient outcome is, "The patient verbalized knowledge of all of their medications and side effects." The six levels from the basic to the most complex are knowledge, comprehension, application, analysis, synthesis and evaluation. Some of the teaching/learning strategies for this domain include online/computer based learning, peer group discussions, reading material and a discussion or lecture.

    Examples of Cognitive Domain Skills for Caregivers:

    Knowledge relating to the signs and symptoms of imminent death, the progression of the end stage disease process, pain and pain management and the importance of properly disposing of medical supplies and equipment.

- *The Psychomotor Domain*

    The psychomotor domain consists of "hands on skills" like taking a blood pressure and using a blood glucose monitor correctly. The seven levels of this domain are perception, set, guided response, mechanism, complex overt response, adaptation and origination. Some of the teaching/learning strategies for this domain include demonstration, return demonstration and a video with a step-by-step demonstration of the psychomotor skill.

    Examples of Psychomotor Domain Skills for Caregivers:

    The administration of pharmacological and non-pharmacological pain interventions, the provision of comfort and hygiene measures and turning and positioning the client

- *The Affective Domain*

    The affective domain includes the development of attitudes, beliefs, values and opinions. An example of affective domain competency is developing a belief that exercise is a valuable part of wellness. The five levels are receiving, responding, valuing, organization and characterization by a value or a value complex. The teaching/learning strategies for this domain include role-playing and values clarification exercises. The affective domain is rarely used for patient teaching.

    Examples of Affective Domain Skills for Caregivers:

    Values clarification in terms of enhancing the client's independence and dignity versus providing total care to the loved one

The Diagnosis of Learning Needs

The diagnosis phase includes the generation of a learning diagnosis based on analyzed assessment data. These diagnosis can include things like "A lack of knowledge about…" and "A knowledge deficit related to…"

Planning Learning Goals and Objectives

The purpose of planning is to ensure that the patient and family teaching is consistent with identified learning needs, and that it can be evaluated in terms of effectiveness (outcome evaluation.) Planning consists of generating objective and specific learning goals, among other things. Learning objectives are specific, measurable, behavioral, learner-centered, consistent with assessed need and congruent with the domain of learning. Examples of well-worded learning objectives are the "Patient will be able to list basic food groups" (cognitive domain) and the "Patient will demonstrate the correct use of a blood glucose monitor" (psychomotor.)

Implementing the Teaching Plan

The implementation phase consists of conducting the education activity in an environment that is conducive to learning, which includes a physically comfortable environment as well as one that is trusting, open, respectful and accepting. Appropriate educational materials, including reading materials are used, as based on the learning needs and the characteristics of the learner, such as sensory impairments and learning styles.

The Evaluation of the Educational Activity

There are two types of evaluation in the teaching/learning process. They are referred to as formative and summative evaluation. Formative evaluation is the continuous assessment of the effectiveness of the teaching while the teaching is being conducted. This allows the teacher to modify the plan, as indicated. Summative evaluation at the end of the learning activity allows the educator to determine whether or not the education has achieved the established learning objectives for the individual or group.

Teaching the Signs and Symptoms of Imminent Death

Hospice and palliative care nurses teach the caregiver and other significant others about the signs and symptoms of imminent death. The primary purpose of this teaching is to allay their fear and to increase their understanding about these signs and symptoms, which can often be distressing and frightening, unless the caregiver understands the underlying perideath process.

Some of these signs and symptoms include body coolness, lethargy, incontinence, confusion, a failure to eat and drink, restlessness, withdrawal and changes in respiratory patterns, including Cheyne-Stokes respirations.

This teaching is within the cognitive domain, therefore, some of teaching strategies include lecture, discussion, reading materials and computer assisted instruction.

Teaching about End-Stage Disease Progression

Caregivers should not only be taught about the progression of the perideath experience, they should also be knowledgeable about the client's specific disease and the progression of this disease. This teaching will facilitate the caregiver's coping skills as well as to enable them to meet and anticipate the ever-changing needs of their loved one.

This teaching is also within the cognitive domain. Therefore, some of teaching strategies include lecture, discussion, reading materials and computer assisted instruction.

Teaching Pain and Symptom Management

Some of this teaching should include the definition of pain, the pain experience, the signs and symptoms of pain and interventions that can be used to increase comfort and decrease pain. Some of these interventions are pharmacological, therefore the caregiver must be knowledgeable about the client's pain medications, the dosage, the frequency and the side effects. Other pain management interventions are non-pharmacological. For these interventions, the caregiver could benefit from education relating to massage therapy, the use of heat and cold and transcutaneous electrical nerve stimulation.

This teaching is within both the cognitive domain and the psychomotor domain. For example, teaching relating to the side effects of medications and the signs of pain are within the cognitive domain. Learning how to perform massage, the use of heat and cold and a TENS machine are within the psychomotor domain of learning. The teaching methods for the cognitive domain include lecture, discussion, reading materials and computer assisted instruction, and the teaching strategies for the psychomotor domain of pain and symptom management can include demonstration, practice time and return demonstration.

Teaching the Benefits and Burdens of Treatment Options

All treatments have benefits and risks; all treatment options and alternatives have to be decided upon by the client, and caregiver as indicated. Under all circumstances, we have the responsibility to educate our clients about these benefits and risks and then allow the client to make an informed decision about whether or not they want the treatment or the alternative. Most times, these decisions are difficult to make, so the hospice and palliative care nurse should assist the client to make decisions based on a sound decision making process.

Decision-making can follow the paternalistic, patient sovereignty or shared decision-making models. Paternalism and patient sovereignty do not respect client autonomy because the clinician makes decisions and the client makes decisions without guidance, respectively. The shared decision-making model upholds client autonomy, because it includes the client, the nurse, and the other members of the healthcare team in a mutually respectful relationship, which enables them to make good decisions with the support of healthcare professionals.

The steps of decision making include:

- Identifying and defining the problem and the purpose of the decision-making. This step often leads to failure when it is not accurate.

- Establishing criteria relating to the desired decision

- Ranking and weighing the criteria in terms of their importance

- Exploring the possible alternatives according to the established criteria

- Deciding on the best alternative as based on the consideration of the potential benefits versus the potential risks

- Making the decision or course of action

- Implementing the decided upon course of action

- Evaluating the outcome of the course of action in terms of its effectiveness

Teaching about Medication Management

Clients at the end of life may have several medications to treat the symptoms of their disease process and the changes at the end of life, including pain management medications. The client and the caregiver should know all about these medications, the dosages, the indications, the side effects and methods of administration.

Teaching about Proper Disposal of Supplies and Equipment

Used needles and other supplies and equipment are biohazardous when they have been contaminated with blood or other bodily fluids. Used needles, and other biohazardous wastes, can transmit diseases, some of which can be life-threatening like hepatitis and HIV/AIDS.

Biohazardous waste can be classified as sharps (needles) and non-sharps like soiled dressings. Soiled dressing and other non-sharp wastes, can be disposed off in community and healthcare settings. Red bags are used for the disposal of biohazardous waste in the healthcare setting. It is recommended that the nurse research disposal practices and regulations in the community so they can provide this important information to their clients.

Disposing of needles or other sharps can be dangerous and pose a health risk to the public. For example, public waste workers can encounter a needle or other sharp if discarded in with the regular trash, and hospital housekeepers can be stuck while cleaning or making a bed.

The U.S. Environmental Protection Agency, in collaboration with the Coalition for Safe Community Needle Disposal, offers solutions for the safe disposal of needles, syringes and other sharps in all areas of the community, including healthcare facilities.

There are several methods for safe disposal:

- *Drop Boxes and Supervised Collection Sites*

    The client may be able to dispose of used needles in community institutions like hospitals, pharmacies, health departments, fire stations, and some doctor's offices.

- *Mail-Back Programs*

    Sharps can also be disposed of by mailing them in a special container to a collection center for a fee.

- *Syringe Exchange Programs (SEP)*

    The North American Syringe Exchange Network provides new needles in exchange for used ones at no cost. The Network may be contacted at (253) 272-4857; its website is www.nasen.org.

- *At-Home Needle Destruction Devices*

    Some products enable in-home destroy needles destruction by severing, burning, or melting the needle, rendering it safer for disposal. An additional alternative in the home includes putting used sharps into a hard container, like an old plastic milk bottle, and disposing of them in their regular trash. Clients should be instructed to contact their solid waste disposal company for specific information relating to sharps disposal.

ADVOCACY

Patient advocacy is a component of practice for nurses. Nurses act in a manner that provides individual clients and groups of clients with the necessary interventions that they need in order to facilitate optimal outcomes. Nurses have a moral and ethical responsibility to enhance clients' decision making autonomy, promote the client's well-being, and prevent and resolve any ethical conflicts.

Monitoring the Need for Changes in Level of Care

Nurses, in collaboration with other members of the healthcare team, don't not only ensure that good care is provided. They must also ensure that the care is provided at the appropriate level.

Levels of care, along the continuum, from the most intensive and expensive to the least, include emergency departments and critical care areas, progressive or "step down" acute care areas, home care and hospice care.

The client's needed level of care depends on a number of factors, including the severity of their disease or disorder, the presence of any complications, the presence of any comorbitities and other factors.

Criteria for admission and discharge from a healthcare facility as well as other levels of care, including hospice and home care, are established by private and governmental agencies, as discussed above. When clients meet admission criteria, the case is accepted and reimbursed for by insurance companies. When a client does not met criteria for admission, the client is referred to another level of care that can be reimbursed by insurance companies.

Hospice and palliative care nurses must ensure that the client is at the appropriate level of care and they must also be able to negotiate with the insurance companies when the nurse, as advocate, often in collaboration with a case manager, believes that a refusal to admit or remain in the same level of care is not in the best interest of the client.

Facilitating Effective Communication

Therapeutic communication enhances the communication process for nurses in their relationships with clients and family members as well as with other members of the health care team.

Some therapeutic communication skills are described below.

- *Seeking Clarification*

Clarification is necessary in order to ensure that the client and the nurse fully understand each other's messages without making any premature or faulty assumptions.

Clarifications can be done with direct and indirect statements and questions, such as "What did you mean about..." or "Tell me more about…."

- *Providing Leads*

Nurses should encourage clients to openly ventilate their feelings and communicate their messages. Providing leads like, "Tell me more about your fears" is lead that is open ended and conducive to client communication.

- *Paraphrasing*

Restating and paraphrasing allows the nurse to acknowledge an understanding about what the client has said and meant in their sent message.

- *Listening*

Active listening is far more than hearing. It is an active process that involves full engagement and a full interpretation of the nonverbal and verbal messages.

- *Praise and Acknowledgment*

Praise and acknowledgement are positive reinforcers that motivate a client to continue moving towards their expected goals.

- *Silence*

The use of therapeutic silence is particularly helpful when the client is expressing deep and profound thoughts, feelings and beliefs that do not necessitate a nurse's response. Prolonged silence, however, may be uncomfortable to the client and may be perceived by the client to be a lack of interest on the part of the nurse.

- *Reflection*

This form of therapeutic communication mirrors the client's feelings, not words, back to the client so they can further explore these feelings with the nurse. For example, when a client expresses anger towards a son because he has not visited for days, the nurse may say, "You seem upset today. Would you like to talk about it?"

- *Perception Validation*

This is similar to clarification in terms of purpose. The nurse, for example, may ask the patient to talk about their feelings and beliefs so the nurse can validate what they perceive they have heard from the client.

- *Offering of Self*

    Nurses offer themselves unconditionally to the client in a compassionate and caring manner.

- *Focusing*

    This form of therapeutic communication enables the client to better focus on and present their main thoughts and ideas so it can be fully understood by the nurse.

- *Summarizing*

    Summarizing is highly useful to sum up the main points of the nurse-client interaction and also to further validate that messages sent and received were interpreted correctly.

All communication should be open, honest and respectful. Group communication and group process communication strategies are discussed below.

Making Referrals

Some interventions can be only carried out by the nurse, while others can be done by other staff with that delegation.

Client care is very complex, and positive outcomes can only be achieved when there is ongoing professional collaboration and cooperation among the many members of the healthcare team as well as financial experts within the facility. In addition to the benefits of collaboration in terms of client care and outcomes, collaboration also enhances commitments, creative problem solving, consensus, and productivity. For example, nurses may collaboratively care for clients to facilitate nutrition in consultation and collaboration with a dietician (diet), a patient educator, a physical therapist, an oncologist, and a social worker to determine the availability of community resources.

Supporting Advance Care Planning

Advance care planning typically consists of a durable power of attorney for health care or health care surrogate, a living will, advance medical care directives and a patient-completed values history. Most often, the advance medical care directive consists of both the living will and the durable power of attorney for health care. Ideally, the client will complete all of these decisions and documents when they are competent and healthy.

Durable Power of Attorney for Healthcare

A durable power of attorney for health care is also called a healthcare proxy or healthcare surrogate. This person is a legally appointed; he or she will make healthcare decisions for the client when the client is no longer competent and able to give legal consent.

Advance Medical Care Directives

Individuals may provide advance medical care directives, or living wills. These specify their treatment wishes—what they do or do not want carried out as part of their care—in the event that they are no longer competent to consent to or reject medical treatment. For example, a young male person with no history of disease may elect to NOT have CPR or a ventilator in the event of sudden death. Another client with cancer may choose to have tube feedings but no IVs in their advanced directive.

The most commonly seen components of advance directives include choices relating to life support measures, mechanical ventilation, intravenous solution administration and methods of artificial feeding, like tube feedings. Many clients at the end of life choose DNR (do not resuscitate), and they specifically state that they do not want mechanical ventilation, intravenous fluids and/or tube feedings.

These directives should be as specific and complete as possible. When an unanticipated event or treatment occurs, that is not included in these advance directive, decisions are made by the durable power of attorney for healthcare in the best interests of the client and their values.

Values Histories

Values histories further support the client's beliefs and opinions in terms of healthcare decisions when they must make decisions, and the living will and durable power of attorney for healthcare needs do not anticipate these decisions. Clients need guidance to make these unanticipated decisions. For example, has the client expressed feelings about life without pain? Has the client expressed beliefs about wanting to die with dignity? Although many healthcare clients do not have a value history, it is highly recommended that nurse help the client to complete one.

Helping the Patient Maintain Optimal Function and Quality of Life

Nurses are obligated to provide comfort and relief of pain for clients in order to help them to maintain optimal function and quality of life.

End-of-life choices are a quality of life issue. Nurses are required to provide medications, aggressive pain relief and control, as well as symptom relief for those at the end of their lives. Nurses are never allowed, however, to administer any medications with the intention of ending a client's life.

Facilitating Self-Determined Life Closure

Hospice and palliative care clients are given thorough assessments, including physically, emotionally, functionally and spiritually at the time of admission. The client or their legal guardian needs to be asked the following two questions:

1. Do you want to avoid hospitalization if your condition worsens?
2. What interventions do you and do you not want at the end of life?

Additionally, advance directives are used to facilitate the client's self-determined life closure.

Monitoring Care for Abuse and Neglect

Abuse and neglect can be physical, psychological, and/or financial. Physical abuse can present as bruises, bone fractures, burns etc. Sexual abuse includes any sexual contact with a minor, or any sexual activity with a person (including spouses) who have not given full consent. Psychological abuse includes actions, such as verbal bullying and threats of harm. Financial abuse can consist of withholding funds from another person.

Examples of neglect are the deprivation of adequate food (physical neglect), isolation and imprisonment in the home (psychological neglect), and a failure to provide another with sufficient funds to purchase things even when there are ample funds to buy it (financial neglect.)

Mandatory Reporting

All states throughout the nation have mandatory reporting laws. Nurses are mandated to report suspected child abuse or neglect, patient abuse or neglect, domestic violence and elder abuse and neglect. Mandated reporters are provided immunity from civil and criminally liability as a result of making a report of any form of abuse, provided that the report was done for valid reason.

VI. INTERDISCIPLINARY AND COLLABORATIVE PRACTICE

SUPERVISION AND DELEGATION

Delegation is the transfer of the nurse's responsibility for the performance of a task to another nursing staff member while retaining accountability for the outcome. Responsibility can be delegated. Accountability CAN NEVER be delegated.

The "Five Rights of Delegation" are:

1. The "right" circumstances
2. The "right" person
3. The "right" task
4. The "right" directions and communication
5. The "right" supervision and evaluation

Proper delegation is crucial in nursing: ineffective and inappropriate delegation can lead to abysmal failures, the lack of goal achievement, illegal practice outside of the scope of practice, and jeopardy of the patient's safety. Delegating responsibilities for patient care to subordinates for whom those duties are beyond their scope of practice puts patients at risk and may even have life-threatening consequences.

In order to ensure high quality care, delegation must be appropriate. It follows that nurses must have an acute knowledge of the healthcare needs of patients; the abilities, competencies, job descriptions, and scope of practice of staff; the law; and policies and procedures.

The Needs of the Client

Successful delegation balances the needs of the patients with abilities of attending staff in accordance with the law and established professional standards.

Those healthcare professionals delegating responsibilities to others must be well-informed about scopes of practice for each of their team members and the standards of care to be upheld. Delegated tasks must be aligned with the delegate's abilities according to the statutory scope of practice, standards of care and practice, and the facility's job description as well as policies and procedures related to the task.

When delegating care, nurses must consider the abilities and competencies of staff members. Each team member is different and unique. When possible, the personal preferences of the patient and the staff member should be accommodated for as long as the delegation is consistent with patient needs, the law, established policies, procedures, job descriptions and the competencies of the individual. The nurse must thoroughly and continuously supervise staff who have been delegated an aspect of care. The delegating nurse is fully accountable for all delegated tasks.

Coordinating Transfers to Different Care Levels and Care Settings

The client's needed level of care depends on a number of factors, including the severity of their disease or disorder, the presence of any comorbitities and other factors. Private health insurance companies and government programs like Medicare and Medicaid establish criteria for admission and discharge to and from a healthcare facility or service, like hospice care.

When the client's needs meet the admission criteria, the case is accepted by the insurance company, including Medicare and Medicaid, and the insurer pays for the admission and service. When a client does not met criteria for admission, the client has to be referred to another level of care. For example, a hospitalized client with terminal cancer may be discharged from an acute care facility when they no longer meet the criteria for acute care; however, they may meet the criteria for a different level of care like home care or hospice care.

Reimbursement is totally dependent on adhering to these established criteria that are based on a number of factors including the hours of nursing care needed, the client's level of independence or dependence, the client's level of functioning and other variables.

Hospice agencies are reimbursed based on the level of care that they provide. The four levels of these services are:

1. Routine home care (RHC)
2. Continuous home care (CHC), which includes a minimum of 8 hours per day for services from a nurse, homemaker or aide, with the priority provider as the RN or LPN/LVN
3. Respite care, which is short-term care on an occasional basis to offer respite and relief to the caregiver and family members. Respite care is reimbursed for up to 5 consecutive days
4. General inpatient care (GIP) when the management of care and symptom relief is not possible in a lesser level of care

COLLABORATION

Collaboration with Care Providers

Collaboration and the coordination of care with other members of the healthcare team were discussed above.

Facilitating Group Process

Some teams are temporary in nature; others are more permanent and ongoing. For example, palliative care and hospice nurses may lead an interdisciplinary case conference for an end of life patient who is highly complex and challenging. The nurse can also participate in an ongoing and permanent Ethics Committee and/or an Oncology Care Committee. All teams, temporary and permanent, go through a growth and development process with relatively predictable challenges and concerns.

The phases of team building, in sequence, are:

1. *Forming*

During this phase of group development, the members of the new group get to know each other and they learn about the mission and purpose of the group. According to Maslow's hierarchy of needs, the members feel a sense of belonging and pride. Typically, the members feel comfortable and friendly, but there is little production and work.

2. *Storming*

Controversies and conflicts arise during this stage. The team members attempt to resolve any conflicts; and, at times, the leadership of the group initiates conflict resolution techniques. Conflict, a naturally occurring event, can be beneficial, but it can also be harmful when it is not recognized and resolved.

3. *Norming*

During the norming phase, the members collectively and collaboratively establish the group's norms and the expectations of its members. Some of these expectations relate to the issue at hand, such as oncology nursing roles, and other expectations related to things like proper behaviors of group members and attendance at meetings.

4. *Performing*

Production and goal achievement are accomplished during this stage. Members are interdependent on other members and they develop some flexibility in terms of their team efforts. Trust is inherent in the group.

5. *Adjourning*

During the adjourning, or mourning, phase the group begins the process of closure. The group has completed their mission; at times, some members can be saddened with this closure. Others may enjoy the closure and experience a sense of accomplishment and self-satisfaction because they played an important role in terms of the group goals.

Evaluating Eligibility for Admission and Hospice Recertification

Appropriate, efficient and consistent healthcare utilization and resource allocation are essential to the provision of care that is driven by medical need and the guidelines and criteria that are established with third party payers, including Medicare and Medicaid.

Utilizing Review Criteria

Using established criteria, relating to medical necessity, nurses should continuously confirm that all clients are at the appropriate level of care and are being provided only those services that are consistent with these established criteria. For this reason, among others, nurses must be highly familiar with these established criteria and have the ability to collaborate and negotiate with members of the healthcare team so that everyone is committed to the importance of efficient and effective care that is consistent with these criteria without compromising quality and positive patient outcomes.

Authorizations

Preadmission insurance authorization, also known as the admission certification, is based on medical necessity. It indicates that the admission of the client to a specific level of care (acute hospital, another inpatient facility, a sub-acute setting, rehabilitation setting) has been deemed appropriate based on the current, documented needs of the client. These authorizations are approved as the direct function of the client's level of acuity, needs and the necessity of medical care at the level that is appropriate.

Medicare, Medicaid and other insurance companies require pre-certification authorizations prior to the rendering of any services or treatments. This initial certification insures a onetime payment based on the patient's diagnosis, which is also known as a diagnosis-related group (DRG) payment.

Concurrent or ongoing authorizations are requested throughout the client's course of care and treatment. These concurrent authorizations are necessary to ensure adequate reimbursement for comorbitities and unanticipated client needs that have occurred since the client was admitted with the pre-certification.

Ideally, and in most cases, the preadmission certification and concurrent authorizations are obtained, but this is not always the case. The third type of authorization is referred to as a pending authorization. This authorization does not ensure reimbursement; it simply indicates that the authorization is being considered. The final decision can be to approve, partially approve, or completely refuse to authorize the care or services.

Denials and Appeals

The best way to avoid the need for appeals is to proactively prevent denials with proactive measures. As the old proverb states, "An ounce of prevention is an equal to a pound of cure." For example, as soon as acute care criteria are no longer met, the client should be discharged or a denial is highly possible; when the length of stay is extended, additional complications and increased disability often occur. This increases costs. Nosocomial infections, falls and skin breakdown are costly beyond the limits of reimbursement. As soon as the nurse learns that reimbursement is not certain, unlikely, or denied, the nurse must act immediately. Some immediate actions include the assessment of the client to determine if there is a medically justified need, and/or the immediate discharge of the client to a more appropriate level of care.

Additional preventive strategies for the nurse include negotiating and communicating with the payer by clearly, objectively and accurately presenting the case and specifically asking the payer which criteria are the basis of their denial or possible denial. If this negotiation is not successful, the nurse must document this discussion and the elements of the discussion and notify the appropriate clinical and administrative staff of this likely denial. The primary reason to document all aspects of this communication is to provide the basis for a future appeal of the denial.

When these preventive measures fail, nurses and other members of the healthcare team play a highly critical and important role in terms of successfully appealing these denials of care. These successes positively affect the reimbursement that the healthcare facility, or hospice care agency, will receive reimbursement for the medically justified care that we provided to the client. Denials have a highly significant effect on the facility's financial status and viability.

The Components of a Successful Appeals Process

The primary purpose of appeals is to recover the costs of provided care and services. A sound and effective appeals process is necessary to recover these costs and to ensure the financial viability of the healthcare organization.

Some of the components of a successful appeals process include:

- *Crystal Clear and Current Payer Criteria*

    Different payers, including Medicare and Medicaid, tend to have similar utilization criteria, but these criteria often change. It is the responsibility of the nurse and other members of the team to continuously remain knowledgeable about these criteria and to be fully informed about any circumstances or situations that could lead to a denial.

- *Establishing and Maintaining Appropriate Contacts*

    One person, or position, must be clearly identified as the contact person that will received communication from payers in terms of possible or actual denials. This one person can be a case manager, a medical billing director, or another appropriate person who will be able to immediately act, either alone or in collaboration, with other members of the organization, such as the job positions mentioned above.

- *Response Mechanisms*

    Organizations must clearly establish response mechanisms to denials. Some of the essential components of these mechanisms are the immediate documentation of this denial, notification of the appropriate designated staff, and actions to respond to the denial in a timely manner. For example, the physician(s) and the nursing case manager should be part of the appeal process. Often, direct communication with the insurer results in the reversal of the denial. Letters to appeal denials must be compelling, based on established criteria, accurate, truthful and detailed.

    Letters of appeal should include the utilization management criteria that the particular insurance company uses, the attending physician, and any authorization numbers that were given by the insurance company during the utilization management interactions with them. The appeal letter should be used to show how the insurance company's criteria match the condition of the patient.

- *Quality Measures*

    Denial data should be tracked and trended over time to prevent future denials. Some of the data that should be collected and analyzed should include the DRG, the lengths of stay, the case type, the provider (physician), the payer, the nursing unit, the nurse caregiver. When trends are analyzed as the aggregate, the variables leading to the denials can be clearly identified so they can be corrected in order to prevent future denials.

- *The Education and Training of Team Members*

    Successful appeals depend on the competency that the members of the appeals team have. Education and training is essential, as is the updating of this knowledge and competency when concerns arise and/or when criteria and processes change.

Some of the commonly occurring denials or non-certifications include partial payments and no-payments for services, support services, durable medical equipment, medications, and increased lengths of stay.

An appeal usually must be filed within thirty to sixty days after the notification of denial. Insurance companies must then reply and respond to the appeal within thirty to sixty days after the appeal is filed. The outcomes of appeals can result in full acceptance and reimbursement, partial acceptance and reimbursement and no acceptance and reimbursement of the appeal. Well designed and implemented appeals processes ensure better success than those that do not possess the above described components.

Encouraging Patient and Family Participation in the Development of an Individualized, Interdisciplinary Plan of Care

As discussed previously, the client is the center of care and they, in addition to significant others, must be actively engaged and involved in all phases of care.

Nurses have a moral and ethical responsibility to enhance clients' decision-making autonomy, the promotion of the client's well being and preventing and resolving any ethical conflicts.

Identifying the Need for Volunteer Services

There are times when volunteers can be highly beneficial to hospice and palliative care clients within the home and within the healthcare facility. Volunteers should be assessed for their suitability in working with a client at the end of life.

Some of the things that volunteers can do include sitting and communicating with the client, providing companionship, reading to the client and helping the person write letters.

Like all members of the healthcare team, volunteers and their roles must be clearly defined in the organization's policies and procedures. Volunteers must have background checks, orientation and training to the organization and their role, as well as the supervision of the professional nurse.

VII. PROFESSIONAL ISSUES

PRACTICE ISSUES

Incorporating Standards into Practice (NHPCO, HPNA, ANA)

The Hospice and Palliative Nurses Association (HPNA) and the American Nursing Association (ANA) have developed an authoritative scope and standards of practice for hospice and palliative care nurses and advanced practice nurses. Even though individual state laws vary, this document articulates the professional standards to which nurses and advanced nurses in palliative and end-of-life care should adhere.

The document specifies that hospice and palliative care nursing seeks to relieve suffering and improve the patient's quality of life throughout the course of the illness, the death of the patient, and the bereavement period of the family. It also discusses education, ethics, advocacy, culture, communication, clinical judgment, professionalism, collaboration, and systems thinking.

You can read more at:

http://www.nursingworld.org/MainMenuCategories/EthicsStandards/Ethics-Position-Statements/etpain14426.pdf

The National Hospice and Palliative Care Organization (NHPCO)

Members of the National Hospice and Palliative Care Organization should subscribe to and practice the following principles:

Internal Relations

Patient and Family

- **Admissions**
  Offer access to hospice and palliative care to all patients and their families in need of those services.

- **Care and Services**
  Provide patients and their families with the highest possible level of quality end-of-life care and services, while maintaining professional boundaries that respect their rights and privacy.

- **Conflicts of Interest**
  Avoid activities that conflict with the organization's responsibilities to patients and their families.

- **Discontinuation of Care**
  Discontinue care only upon the voluntary consent of the patient, when the patient is no longer medically eligible, or when the organization cannot provide care without compromising the ethical or professional integrity, or the safety, of its employees.

- **Information Management, Confidentiality and Privacy**
  Respect and protect confidential information.

Employees and Volunteers

- **Employee and Volunteer Relations**
  Ensure that hospice and palliative care employees and volunteers are treated with respect and fairness, while supporting their ability to obtain the highest level of skill and expertise in their profession or role.

Governance

- **Governance**
  Adhere to governance structures that ensure the organization fulfills its mission and purpose.

External Relations

Hospice Market (other hospices, suppliers, payers)

- **External Collegial Relationships**
  Work cooperatively with other healthcare providers, suppliers and payers to provide compassionate and competent end-of-life care.

Donors

- **Development and Fundraising**
  Be open and transparent in soliciting and accepting financial and/or in-kind support

General Public

- **Access**
  Promote universal availability of comprehensive hospice and palliative care services, in diverse healthcare settings and with specific emphasis on reaching traditionally underserved populations.

- **Marketing and Referrals**
  Follow marketing and referral practices that promote compassionate, high-quality care for patients and their families.

- **Public Information**
  Develop and disseminate accurate, honest and timely information about hospice, palliative care and other end-of-life issues to local, state and national communities.

Society

- **Research**
  Support the advancement of knowledge to improve the provision, quality, and outcomes of hospice and palliative care."[1]

Preamble and Philosophy

"Hospice affirms the concept of palliative care as an intensive program that enhances comfort and promotes the quality of life for individuals and their families. When cure is no longer possible, hospice recognizes that a peaceful and comfortable death is an essential goal of health care. Hospice believes that death is an integral part of the life cycle and that intensive palliative care focuses on pain relief, comfort and enhanced quality of life as appropriate goals for the terminally ill. Hospice also recognizes the potential for growth that often exists within the dying experience for the individual and his/her family and seeks to protect and nurture this potential.

Terminal illness is frequently defined as the point where nothing more can be done to cure someone. This limited focus and lack of concern for caring issues such as pain and symptom control can lead to increased suffering and isolation for patients and family members. In reality, supportive, positive care directed toward comfort and growth can be offered to individuals and their families during the end of life.

Hospice addresses the needs and opportunities during the last phase of life by including the individual and family, trained volunteers, caregivers and clinical professionals in the care giving team. This interdisciplinary approach to care focuses on the individual's physical symptoms and the emotional and spiritual concerns of the patient and family. The team works together to develop a plan of care and to provide services that will enhance the quality of life and provide support for the individual and family while respecting their wishes during the terminal phases of the illness and the bereavement period."[2]

Hospice Philosophy Statement

"Hospice provides support and care for persons in the last phases of an incurable disease so that they may live as fully and as comfortably as possible. Hospice recognizes that the dying process is a part of the normal process of living and focuses on enhancing the quality of

---

[1] "Ethical Principles," National Hospice and Palliative Care Organization, accessed October 20, 2015, http://www.nhpco.org/ethical-principles.
[2] "Preamble to NHPCO Standards of Practice," National Hospice and Palliative Care Organization, accessed October 20, 2015, http://www.nhpco.org/ethical-and-position-statements/preamble-and-philosophy.

remaining life. Hospice affirms life and neither hastens nor postpones death. Hospice exists in the hope and belief that through appropriate care, and the promotion of a caring community sensitive to their needs that individuals and their families may be free to attain a degree of satisfaction in preparation for death. Hospice recognizes that human growth and development can be a lifelong process. Hospice seeks to preserve and promote the inherent potential for growth within individuals and families during the last phase of life. Hospice offers palliative care for all individuals and their families without regard to age, gender, nationality, race, creed, sexual orientation, disability, diagnosis, availability of a primary caregiver, or ability to pay.

Hospice programs provide state-of-the-art palliative care and supportive services to individuals at the end of their lives, their family members and significant others, 24 hours a day, seven days a week, in both the home and facility-based care settings. Physical, social, spiritual, and emotional care is provided by a clinically-directed interdisciplinary team consisting of patients and their families, professionals, and volunteers during the:

1. Last stages of an illness;
2. Dying process; and
3. Bereavement period.

The National Hospice and Palliative Care Organization (NHPCO) defines palliative care as treatment that enhances comfort and improves the quality of an individual's life during the last phase of life. No specific therapy is excluded from consideration. The test of palliative care lies in the agreement between the individual, physician(s), primary caregiver, and the hospice team that the expected outcome is relief from distressing symptoms, the easing of pain, and/or the enhancing the quality of life. The decision to intervene with active palliative care is based on an ability to meet stated goals rather than affect the underlying disease. An individual's needs must continue to be assessed and all treatment options explored and evaluated in the context of the individual's values and symptoms. The individual's choices and decisions regarding care are paramount and must be followed at all times."[3]

http://www.nhpco.org/ethical-and-position-statements/preamble-and-philosophy

The American Nurses Association's Standards of Practice and Standards of Care

The American Nurses Association's Standards of Practice and Standards of Care include the following fifteen (15) competencies that are expected of all nurses, including hospice and palliative care nurses:

1. Assessment
2. Diagnosis
3. Outcomes evaluation
4. Planning

---

[3] "Preamble to NHPCO Standards of Practice," National Hospice and Palliative Care Organization, accessed October 20, 2015, http://www.nhpco.org/ethical-and-position-statements/preamble-and-philosophy.

5. Implementation
6. Evaluation
7. Quality of practice
8. Education
9. Professional practice evaluation
10. Collegiality
11. Collaboration
12. Ethics
13. Research
14. Resource utilization
15. Leadership

The American Nurses Association's Code of Ethics

The American Nurses Association's Code of Ethics, like the American Nurses Association's Standards of Practice and Standards of Care, apply to all nurses in all diverse roles and in all healthcare settings. This Code emphasizes the dignity and worth of all people without discrimination, the nurses' commitment to patients, advocacy, accountability, the preservation of safety, patient rights, such as dignity, autonomy and confidentiality, competency, the provision of quality care, collaboration, the integrity of the nursing profession and the resolution of ethical dilemmas and/or conflicts.

Ethical Principles

Some of the ethical principles that nurses must adhere to during all aspects of nursing care and practice are:

- *Justice:*

    The principle of justice requires us to be fair to all. For example, limited resources must be fairly and justly distributed among patients.

- *Fidelity*

    Fidelity is being faithful to one's promises. The nurse-client relationship implies that the nurse follows through on professional promises and responsibilities by providing high quality, safe care in a competent, scientifically grounded manner while upholding the clients' choices, desires and innate rights.

- *Beneficence*

    Although beneficence may appear to be the opposite of non-maleficence, it is not. Beneficence simply stated means "Do good." Doing "good" is more than just not doing any harm (non-maleficence.) On occasions, beneficence can lead to unanticipated harm. For example, when a nurse administers an ordered medication and it leads to side effects, these side effects are considered an unanticipated side effect or unanticipated harm.

- *Non-maleficence*

Non-maleficence is "Do not harm", as stated in the Hippocratic Oath. Harm can be intentional or unintentional, as is the case when a client has an adverse effect to a medication, such as a chemotherapy drug. For obvious reasons, intentional harm is much more serious than unintentional harm.

- *Accountability*

All nurses are accountable for all aspects of nursing care. They must answer to themselves, their clients and society for their actions and they must accept any, and all, personal and professional consequences for all of their actions.

- *Autonomy and Self Determination*

Each unique individual has the right to make choices without coercion or the undue influence of others. All nurses never impose their own beliefs, values or opinions on the client. They accept all client choices without any judgments. The patient has the right to choose and/or refuse any and all treatments or interventions.

- *Veracity*

Veracity is truthfulness. Nurses do not withhold the whole truth from clients even when it may be upsetting or distressful to the client.

All nurses must demonstrate ethical competency with patient advocacy, holding themselves accountable for practice, mediating ethical conflicts and dilemmas, responding to ethical problems, and critically evaluating changes and technologies in terms of clients' well being and ethical principles.

INCORPORATING GUIDELINES INTO PRACTICE

National Guideline Clearinghouse and the Agency for Healthcare Research and Quality

The National Guideline Clearinghouse and the Agency for Healthcare Research and Quality (AHRQ) have collectively developed a highly extensive database of evidence-based clinical practice guidelines and related documents. These guidelines are updated every week and, at the moment, there are 56 practice guidelines for hospice care alone. These guidelines can be accessed at:

http://www.guideline.gov/search/search.aspx?term=hospice

The National Consensus Project

The National Consensus Project and the National Quality Forum together have developed eight domains of palliative care. These domains include:

1. Structure and Processes of Care
2. Physical Aspects of Care
3. Psychological and Psychiatric Aspects of Care
4. Social Aspects of Care
5. Spiritual, Religious and Existential Aspects of Care
6. Cultural Aspects of Care
7. Care of the Imminently Dying Patient
8. Ethical and Legal Aspects of Care

The most current complete edition, including the specific guidelines for each domain, can be accessed at:

http://www.nationalconsensusproject.org/GuidelinesTOC.pdf

INCORPORATING LEGAL REGULATIONS INTO PRACTICE

The Health Insurance Portability and Accountability Act (HIPAA)

The Health Insurance Portability and Accountability Act (HIPAA) protects a patient's right to maintain the privacy and confidentiality of all his or her oral, written, and electronic medical information, unless the patient has provided express written consent to its disclosure. Access to all, or part, of the medical record is restricted to only those who have a "need to know". Many of those who have the "right to know and the need to know" are those who provide direct care to the patient; others who also have the legal "need to know" are those that provide indirect care and reimbursement. For example, a physical therapist, insurance companies, the case manager or a QA nurse may have a need to know even when they are not providing direct care to the patient because of the nature of their role.

Implications for the nurse in terms of HIPAA are numerous and the penalties for violations are severe. Some of the implications include prohibitions against discussing patients with others who do not have the "need to know", protecting patient's written records and logging off after accessing electronic medical records. Idle discussions about patients in the community, in the hospital elevator and/or cafeteria are prohibited; telephone conversations with unknown people without a code, or other unique identifier, are prohibited; logging off the computer and securing a hard copy chart so others cannot view them is mandatory; Facebook discussions and cell phone pictures are strictly prohibited.

Omnibus Budget Reconciliation Act (OBRA)

The Omnibus Budget Reconciliation Act (OBRA) of 1987, also referred to as the Federal Nursing Home Reform Act, established regulations for nursing homes, which have to be strictly adhered to in order for nursing homes to receive federal and state reimbursement from Medicaid and Medicare for services rendered to residents.

The primary foci of these regulations include the roles, training, certification, continuing education and competencies of certified nursing assistants. The states, according to OBRA, can develop and implement their own basic training and education programs. However, this education must be a minimum of at least 75 hours with at least 16 hours of clinical training that is supervised by the nurse and other classroom content that includes topics like infection control, respect and dignity and communication skills.

The states regulate the certified nursing assistant and certify nursing assistants, and they also administer the state's clinical and knowledge aspects of the certified nursing assistant examination.

The United States Department of Labor Occupational Safety and Health Administration (OSHA)

OSHA has regulations that protect healthcare workers. These regulations focus on infection control, standard precautions, personal protective equipment such as eye, face, and respiratory protective devices, ionizing radiation, chemicals, sharps safety and other protections.

Centers for Medicare and Medicaid Services

In addition to the information about Medicare and Medicaid requirements and reimbursement that was discussed previously, fraud is a serious legal offense that has serious legal consequences. Compliance officers strive to prevent breaches of the False Claims Act such as billing for services not provided, kickbacks, and billing for substandard care. Fraud and abuse can occur in all aspects of care and in all levels of care.

"Whistle blower", or Qui Tam provisions, protect those that report violations. Additionally, organizations have duty to report all overpayments. Thorough documentation is one way to prevent fraud and abuse.

Educating the Public on End of Life and Palliative Care

Among other roles and responsibilities, hospice and palliative care nurses have the professional responsibility to market hospice and palliative care as well as educate the public about it and its benefits.

Evaluating Educational Materials

In addition to evaluating overall staff and patient education programs and individual educational activities in terms of effectiveness, educational materials for patients and family members are also evaluated. Some of the things that you should consider include:

- Were the educational materials complete and appropriate to the domain of learning?
- Were the educational materials accurate, current and effective in terms of meeting the clients' learning needs?
- Were the educational materials culturally sensitive, understandable, and at the appropriate reading level when written materials are used?

Conflict Management

Conflicts are a natural part of all interactions. Conflicts can be intrapersonal (ethical or moral concerns), interpersonal, and organizational (interdepartmental conflicts.) Conflicts cannot be avoided and they often lead to beneficial changes. Most conflicts can be resolved in a beneficial manner; however some just cannot be resolved. Conflicts arise when there are disparate opinions, values, beliefs and attitudes.

Nurses must be skilled in terms of conflict resolution. The best ways to resolve conflicts is to have the group discuss their beliefs and attitudes, and then negotiate a resolution, with the guidance of the nurse. Conflicts can, and should be, resolved with negotiation and compromise whenever possible. Coercion does not solve conflicts in a beneficial manner. Collective communication and collaboration does.

Evidence-Based Practice

Evidence-based practice is research-based practice. Simply stated, evidence-based practice begins with research, and then this research is applied to the development of evidence-based practice guidelines which are disseminated through a wide variety mechanisms, including publications and professional conferences. These evidence-based practice guidelines can and should be applied to practice after the research and guidelines are critiqued by the nurse.

Some areas of consideration for integrating evidence-based practices into one's role as a hospice, palliative care nurse include:

- Is the evidence-based practice feasible and practical?
- Do the potential benefits of the evidence-based practice outweigh the possible risks and costs associated with its implementation?
- Is it potentially effective and efficient or is it too time consuming and limited in terms of effectiveness?

Providing an evidence-based approach to care requires that the nurse can:

- Access and appraise evidence (research findings)
- Understand the relationships between research and the strength of evidence
- Determine its applicability in respect to a particular patient's condition, context and wishes.

Critiques relating to the evidence-based practice guidelines include:

- the date of the publication
- the author(s)
- the basis of the guideline in terms of whether or not research was used
- the quality of the comprehensive reference list
- the professional organization that endorses the guideline
- the review of the guidelines by an expert, or expertly, in the field of practice being addressed
- whether the guideline has been successfully utilized in practice with optimal outcomes.

Some of the databases that nurses can use regularly to review research and evidence-based practice are listed below along with the correlate internet link:

- The Cochrane Library
  http://www.thecochranelibrary.com/view/0/AboutTheCochraneLibrary.html

- The Joanna Briggs Institute
  http://www.joannabriggs.edu.au/

- Ovid's Evidence-based Medicine Reviews (EBMR)
  http://www.ovid.com/webapp/wcs/stores/servlet/ProductDisplay?storeId=13051&catalogId=13151&langId=-1&partNumber=Prod-904410

- Medlars
  http://www.nlm.nih.gov/bsd/mmshome.html

- Medline Plus (An International nursing index and Index Medicus is also included)
  http://www.nlm.nih.gov/medlineplus/

- Pub Med
  http://www.ncbi.nlm.nih.gov/pubmed/

- The Cumulative Index to Nursing and Allied Health Literature (CINAHL)
  http://www.ebscohost.com/cinahl/)

- The Directory of Open Access Journals (Free)
  http://www.doaj.org

- The Nursing Center for Lippincott Williams & Wilkins'
  http://nursingcenter.com

Educating Health Care Providers Regarding Medicare and Medicaid Hospice Benefits

Again, the hospice and palliative care nurse should educate others, including other healthcare providers, about hospice and palliative care, its purposes and its benefits to the client and significant others, and also about the reimbursement for these services under Medicare and Medicaid, as discussed above.

Quality Assurance and Performance Improvement

Measuring quality has evolved over the years from quality control, to quality assurance, quality improvement to performance improvement, and continuous quality improvement. It has also evolved from structure studies, to process studies, to outcome-related studies. Successful quality management and performance improvement activities improve the outcomes of care and the safety and efficiency of processes and reduce costs, risks and liability.

These activities are mandated by external regulatory bodies such as the Joint Commission on the Accreditation of Healthcare Organizations (JCAHO), the Centers for Medicare and Medicaid (CMS) and state departments of health. Quality management is an integral part of the nurse's role, as well as an integral part of every healthcare provider's responsibility. Efforts should focus on areas with the greatest risk, the greatest volume, the highest costs and the most problem prone.

Although models differ somewhat, continuous quality, or performance, improvement activities include the identification of an opportunity to improve a process, organizing a team to work on the improvement activity (those closely related to the process must be included in the group), identifying client expectations and outcomes, gathering data and information, including best practices and research studies, and analyzing the data. It also includes the close examination of the existing process, designing the process with measurable specifications that can be evaluated, the elimination of all variances, the implementation of the newly designed process, the evaluation of improvement in terms of the measurable specifications, and a thorough documentation of the entire procedure that led to the process change.

Some of the critical aspects of palliative and hospice care that should be evaluated with quality and performance improvement include client safety, the effectiveness of processes and systems in terms of error prevention and reduction and the timeliness of care. Other aspects include the efficiency of care, the appropriateness of care, the effectiveness of care, the patient centeredness of care, and the ethics of care (accessibility to care and equitable care, etc.)

All domains of palliative and hospice care nursing should be addressed with quality assessment studies. For example, the structure and process relating to the overall hospice program, the utilization of team members, educational activities, ethical actions, and effectiveness of physical, psychological, psychiatric, social, spiritual, and cultural aspects of care can be explored. Studies should be multidisciplinary.

Quality Indicators

Quality indicators can be categorized as core measures and outcome measures. Core measures are standardized measures of quality. JCAHO has ORYX National Hospital Quality Measures that include disease-related measures, such as cancer, population measures, such as pediatric care, and organizational measures, like those used in the oncology area.

Structure, processes and outcomes can be evaluated with data. Data can be quantitative or qualitative. For example, the prevalence or incidence of falls and nosocomial infections are examples of quantitative data. Patient satisfaction and quality of life are often anecdotal narrative comments. This data is considered qualitative data although these two anecdotal levels can also be quantified using a quantitative measurement scale or tool so they can be analyzed and evaluated with quantitative statistical analysis.

Outcomes will be unpredictable and filled with variances if the process and the structure are not stable. Unstable structures and processes will lead to unstable outcomes. The goal is to achieve and maintain stable and predictably high quality outcomes, so good structures and processes must be in place and concretized before outcomes can be stabilized, improved and optimized.

Nurses can, and should, measure outcomes relating to physiological or biological health problems, psychological measures, infection rates after surgery, MRSA rates, patient satisfaction findings, lengths of stay, readmissions, quality of life, functional abilities, goal attainment, safety, and the occurrence of adverse events.

These measurements can also involve the measurement of performance over time in a longitudinal manner to determine if planned changes have sustained increased performance, and to identify problems and opportunities for improvement.

National Patient Safety Goals

The purpose of the National Patient Safety Goals is to improve patient safety. The goals focus on problems in health care safety and how to solve them. The Joint Commission on the Accreditation of Healthcare Organization (JCAHO) publishes these goals on an annual basis.

The hospital Patient Safety Goals for 2013 include the goals to:

- Identify patients correctly
- Prevent infection
- Improve staff communication
- Identify patient safety risks
- Prevent mistakes in surgery
- Use medications correctly

More information about Patient Safety Goals can be seen at the following link: http://www.jointcommission.org/standards_information/npsgs.aspx

Risk Management

Risk management is closely aligned with continuous quality improvement, but instead of proactively planning change like quality improvement, risk management aims to identify and reduce liability by eliminating risks and liabilities that can include client related risks, quality risks, and financial risks and liabilities.

Nurses must be able to identify patients who are vulnerable to high-risk incidents. For example, all patients should be screened for falls risk, infection risk, and skin breakdown. Immediate and specific preventive measures are put in place for all "at risk" clients. Risk management identifies and eliminates hazards relating to basic safety, such as falls, elopement, and infant abduction, a wide variety of medical errors, such as wrong site surgery, wrong patient surgery and medication errors. JCAHO has requirements relating to medical errors in terms of reporting sentinel events and the elimination of hazards using root cause analysis.

Safety and Risk Management Considerations

Nurses are responsible and accountable for the safety of clients, significant others, visitors and all staff who are in the healthcare setting. Some of these potential safety needs and concerns include:

- Internal and external disasters
- Falls and other events like elopement of clients and abduction of infants
- Infections
- Biohazardous waste and sharps management

Root Cause Analysis

Root cause analysis is a process that is used to dig down to the deepest, real reasons why mistakes and errors have occurred. These reasons are usually procedures and processes and NOT people. Root cause analysis occurs in a blame- free environment with teams of stakeholders who closely analyze faulty processes with a number of techniques such as brain storming, flow charting, fishbone diagrams, data collection and statistical data analysis.

It is recommended that all sentinel events are examined using root cause analysis. A sentinel event is an occurrence that leads to, or has the potential to lead to, an adverse outcome. For example, when a client has a left leg amputation instead of a right leg amputation, it leads to liability and actual harm. On the other hand, when a nurse is about to administer an incorrect medication or dosage and they suddenly realize that they are about to err and they stop and correct the dosage it is also a sentinel event. Even "near-misses" are considered sentinel events.

The processes that actually cause harm as well as those that lead to "near-misses" must be refined and improved so that all possible human errors are eliminated and future sentinel events can be prevented.

Some of the most commonly occurring medical error sentinel events include the unintended retention of a foreign body after surgery or another invasive procedure, wrong patient/wrong site/ wrong procedure, treatment delays, suicide, operative and post operative complications, falls, criminal events, medication errors, perinatal death and other unanticipated events.

Variance Tracking

There are four types of variance including practitioner variance, system/institutional variance, community variance and patient/family variances. In the context of continuous quality improvement, a variance is a quality defect.

Variances can be random and they can be specific. A random variance is one that occurs because of things inherent to the process; these variances occur each time the established process is carried out. Specific variances occur because of one specific part of the process. Both of these variances indicate that efforts must be made to correct and eliminate variance.

Benchmarking and Best Practices

Benchmarking and the identification of best practices are superior ways that quality and risk can be objectively determined. Some hospitals provide care that is less costly than others; some hospitals achieve better client outcomes than others; and some hospitals have lower incidences of sentinel events than others. Nurses should identify these best practices and attempt to replicate these best practices so they can continuously improve quality.

Data Management

Data can be collected and analyzed to measure outcomes both in terms of an individual and it can be collected and analyzed to measure outcomes in terms of a group, population or aggregate. For example, a hospice or palliative care nurse may use data to measure the effectiveness of a program, like a hospice palliative care program, or the outcomes of care for aggregated populations, such as the outcomes of care for a population of clients who are affected with cancer, severe depression, and end of life symptoms.

Electronic Medical Records

All medical records are legal documents. Documentation must be complete, timely, accurate and professional. The purposes of documentation include communication among members of the healthcare team, to fulfill the legal requirements of Medicare's Conditions of Participation and reimbursement, and to fulfill the mandates of external regulatory bodies, such as Joint Commission on the Accreditation of Healthcare Organizations and the state departments of health.

Good documentation facilitates optimal and timely communication among team members, complete and appropriate care, timeliness of care, the prevention of errors of omission, commission and duplication, and the minimization of treatment delays. The characteristics of good documentation include legibility, accuracy, completeness, timeliness and done in a professional manner. It must be clear, understandable, and without errors.

Most documentation errors are errors of omission. The nurse fails to document something that should have been documented. Other documentation errors are errors of commission. For example, the nurse may document faulty assessment data that was related to one of the nurse's other patients. All documentation errors can lead to serious patient related consequences including death.

Some of the things that the nurse must do in order to legally and completely document include ensuring that the chart has the correct name before entering information into it, writing legibly, accurately dating and timing the entry and ending all entries with a full signature and title. They also include correcting errors by placing a thin line through the erroneous entry and printing the word "error" above it with your signature, and entering documentation as soon as possible after care is rendered and/or new data is available without any "pre charting." Additionally, under no circumstances should a nurse document for anyone else, and documentation must be professional in terms of grammar, spelling, punctuation and objectivity. Documentation must be objective and free of judgments like "the patient is rude or uncooperative."

The most commonly used documentation methods are listed below. All of these methods have their unique advantages and disadvantages.

- Source oriented medical record
- Problem oriented medical record
- Focus charting
- Charting by exception
- Case management/critical pathways

All medical records can be electronic or hard copy. When electronic medical records are used, it is important that you not share your user name and password with others and that you log off the computer when you are done with your entry in order to ensure the client's right to the privacy and confidentiality of their medical information.

All hospitals and other healthcare settings, such as hospice centers, vary in terms of which records are electronic and what computer software is used to generate and maintain these records. Nurses must be competent in the navigation and use of these various electronic records.

PROFESSIONAL DEVELOPMENT

Contributing to Professional Development

All nurses, including hospice and palliative care nurses, have a professional responsibility to mentor and precept others new to the profession, new to hospice and palliative care and/or new to the organization.

Resolving Ethical Concerns Related to the End of Life

Ethical dilemmas and conflicts are on the rise because of a number of factors, including the wide variety and diversity of treatment options and the ongoing debate about who should get limited resources.

Nurses must identify sources of ethical conflict and initiate changes to avoid them in the future. Many healthcare facilities have multidisciplinary ethics committees that convene to resolve ethical dilemmas and conflicts. Ideally, the members of this committee have had some advanced training and education relating to bioethics to maximize their ability to provide guidance in respect to ethical dilemmas and conflicts.

Some of the commonly occurring ethical dilemmas that affect clients revolve around euthanasia, physician assisted suicide, the continued administration of pain medications to relieve pain even when it hastens death, advance directives and withholding food and fluids.

Participating in Peer Review

Peer review is another strategy that can be used to identify opportunities for improvement. With this type of review, peers, such as certified hospice and palliative care nurses, collaboratively work together to critically evaluate aspects of care.

Maintaining Professional Boundaries

According to the Life Quality Institute's Advancing Palliative Care, professional boundaries are the lines that separate the client from the nurse, or another healthcare professional. Professional boundaries ensure safe, professional and appropriate interactions despite the fact that the client, as the vulnerable person, and the nurse, as the person in "power", are dynamically interacting.

Professional boundaries can be violated intentionally and unintentionally when the limits of this therapeutic relationship are crossed even when it leads to no client harm. Some examples of actions that violate professional boundaries include accepting gifts from clients, a nurse's sharing of personal information, calling clients with names such as "mom" or "honey", unprofessional demeanor and an excessive and/or inappropriate use of touch.

For more information about professional boundaries, go to
http://www.capnm.ca/Prof_Boundaries_Packet_2010.pdf

Stress Management

Nurses have the professional and personal responsibility to care for themselves. This includes measures to ensure and maintain optimal physical and mental health. For example, nurses should have an annual physical, complete and current immunization status, including the influenza and pneumonia vaccine, healthy lifestyle choices and psychological health and wellness.

Nursing is a stressful job, so nurses must also be able to manage their stress using the same nonpharmacological stress management techniques that they use with and for their clients such as exercise, yoga, meditation, progressive relaxation, prayer, imagery, deep breathing, and distraction.

Staying Current on Medical and Nursing Literature

Nurses are accountable for their own personal competency and current knowledge. Although many nurses believe that continuing education consists of only formal educational activities, continuing education also consists of reading medical and nursing literature to update and upgrade one's knowledge and skills.

Some of the journals that are useful to palliative care and hospice care nurses are the American Journal of Nursing, the American Nurse Today, Cancer Nursing, the Clinical Journal of Oncology Nursing, Evidence-based Nursing, Journal of the American Geriatrics Society, the Journal of Hospice and Palliative Nursing and the Online Journal of Issues in Nursing. Others include the Oncology Nursing Forum, Pain Management Nursing, the Journal of Hospice and Palliative Nursing and the American Journal of Hospice and Palliative Medicine.

Participating in Nursing Associations

Hospice and palliative care nurses should participate in nursing associations such as The Hospice and Palliative Nurses Association, the National Association of Homecare and Hospice, the National Hospice and Palliative Care Organization, the American Nurses Association, and the state Boards of Nursing.

Continuing Education

As stated above, continuing education and current knowledge is the professional responsibility of all nurses including those who are working in hospice and palliative care. Continuing education and enhanced knowledge facilitate quality client care and it is also mandated by some states for license renewal as well as the National Board for Certification of Hospice and Palliative Nurses for CHPN recertification if the examination is not retaken.

Staying Current on Laws and Policies

Hospice and palliative care nurses should be involved in public policy making and legislative issues, as well as running for public office. These nurses can be the best advocates for issues, such as Medicare and Medicaid reimbursement, the accessibility and affordability of hospice and palliative care services, and some of the ethical and legal issues at the end of life including physician assisted suicide and advance directives.

VIII. PRACTICE QUESTIONS

1. It is most difficult to predict the time of death and life expectancy when the disease process:

   A. Abruptly threatens life
   B. Deteriorates rapidly
   C. Has a sudden onset
   D. Is chronic and prolonged

2. What are the three phases of the perideath process in correct sequential order?

   A. Preparation for death, the death itself and after death
   B. Onset, peak, duration and death
   C. Preparation for death, onset of symptoms and death
   D. Onset, duration, peak and death

3. Which of the following is a sign or symptom of the first phase of perideath?

   A. Fever
   B. Intermittent hunger
   C. Intermittent thirst
   D. Withdrawal

4. Select the disorder that is accurately paired with its description.

   A. Disseminated intravascular coagulation: A primary condition or disorder that affects only clotting factors
   B. Hypocalcemia: A disorder that commonly affects clients with bone, lung and breast cancer
   C. Increased intracranial pressure: A cerebral disorder that results from a intracranial pressure of greater than 3
   D. Thrombotic thrombocytopenia purpura: A clotting disorder that affects vessels throughout the body

5. Which type of shock is your client at greatest risk for as the result of an indwelling urinary catheter?

   A. Neurogenic shock
   B. Septic shock
   C. Anaphylactic shock
   D. Hypovolemic shock

6. Select the stage of hypovolemic shock that is correctly paired with its symptom.

   A. Initial stage: Metabolic acidosis
   B. Secondary stage: Respiratory acidosis
   C. Compensatory stage: Vasodilation
   D. Progressive stage: Decreased urinary output

7. Which client is at greatest risk for spinal cord compression?

   A. A 26 year old male client with lymphoma
   B. A 56 year old post-menopausal woman
   C. An 86 year old male with primary cancer of the testes
   D. A 35 year old with disseminated intravascular coagulation

8. Your oncology client has facial and periorbital edema, respiratory distress, and cyanosis. Which disorder is this client most likely affected with?

   A. Acites
   B. Increased intracranial pressure
   C. Vena cava syndrome
   D. Cardiac tamponade

9. Your client has a nursing diagnosis of "Activity intolerance r/t an oxygen demand that is greater than the oxygen supply". Which disorder is this client most likely affected with?

   A. Pneumonitis
   B. Chronic obstructive pulmonary disease
   C. Pneumothorax
   D. Vena cava syndrome

10. Which fact about urinary tract infections is accurate?

    A. Males are at greater risk for urinary tract infections than females
    B. Females are at less risk for urinary tract infections than males
    C. Klebsiella is the most common pathogen associated with urinary tract infections
    D. Indwelling urinary catheters place clients at risk for urinary tract infections

11. Which content should be included in a client teaching plan about urinary tract infections?

    A. The need to drink at least 3 liters of fluid per day when a urinary tract infection is present
    B. The need to drink at least 2 liters of fluid per day when a urinary tract infection is present
    C. The importance of using only synthetic fiber under pants to prevent a urinary tract infection
    D. The importance of drinking diet drinks with aspartame rather than other sweeteners

12. Your client is excreting 246 mg of albumin in 24 hours. What is causing this excretion amount?

    A. Abnormal hepatic functioning
    B. Normal hepatic functioning
    C. Abnormal renal functioning
    D. Normal renal functioning

13. Your client will be having a Billroth II surgical procedure. What should the nurse include in this client's teaching plan?

    A. Things, including foods, which can increase vitamin A
    B. Things, including foods, which can increase calcium levels
    C. Dumping syndrome signs and symptoms
    D. The effect of a Billroth II in the palliation of peptic ulcers

14. Odynophagia is defined as:

    A. Difficulty swallowing
    B. Substernal chest pain
    C. Esophageal varices
    D. Impaired sensory function

15. Which fact about pancreatic cancer is accurate?

    A. The prognosis is poor because it is often asymptomatic in its early stages
    B. A pancreatoduodenectomy is highly effective for most clients
    C. Those over 70 years of age are at greatest risk for it
    D. Most pancreatic cancers form at the tail of the pancreas

16. Which type of cancer is most likely to metastasize to the liver?

    A. Cancer of the breast
    B. Cancer of the brain
    C. Hodgkin's disease
    D. Leukemia

17. Select the form of nutrition that is correctly paired with its side effect or indication.

    A. Enteral nutrition: Diarrhea
    B. Enteral nutrition: This form of nutrition is indicated when the anticipated duration of nutritional support is less than 4 weeks
    C. Parenteral nutrition: Diarrhea
    D. Parenteral nutrition: This form of nutrition is indicated when the anticipated duration of nutritional support is less than 4 weeks

18. Your client is irritable, has lost interest in life and is avoiding eye contact. Which disorder is this client most likely affected with?

    A. Disuse syndrome
    B. Malabsorption
    C. Failure to thrive
    D. Death anxiety

19. Which disorder is characterized with steatorrhea and explosive diarrhea?

    A. Failure to thrive
    B. Dumping syndrome
    C. Disuse syndrome
    D. Malabsorption

20. A major difference between delirium and dementia is that delirium is:

    A. Typically has a slow onset and dementia does not
    B. Persistent for less than 3 days and dementia lasts longer
    C. Is typically progressive until unconsciousness occurs
    D. Sometimes reversible and dementia is not

21. Which fact about the syndrome of inappropriate antidiuretic hormone secretion is accurate?

    A. The syndrome of inappropriate antidiuretic hormone secretion is a metabolic endocrine disorder
    B. The syndrome of inappropriate antidiuretic hormone secretion is associated with spinal cord injuries
    C. The syndrome of inappropriate antidiuretic hormone secretion places clients at risk of cerebral edema
    D. The syndrome of inappropriate antidiuretic hormone secretion presents with increased sodium excretion and hyper-osmolality

22. As you are caring for a client with type 2 diabetes, the client expresses concerns about the acute complications of diabetes. What should you teach this client about?

    A. The role of good blood glucose control in terms of preventing hyperglycemic hyperosmolar nonketotic coma
    B. The role of good blood glucose control in terms of preventing neuropathy and nephropathy
    C. The role of regular exercise in terms of preventing peripheral neuropathy
    D. The role of regular exercise in terms of preventing diabetic retinopathy

23. You have completed a full assessment of your client. You will now be establishing priorities. What phase of the nursing process includes establishing priorities?

    A. Diagnosing
    B. Priority setting
    C. Planning
    D. Implementation

24. You are reviewing your client's recent laboratory results. What type of data is this?

    A. Objective, secondary data
    B. Objective, primary data
    C. Subjective, empirical data
    D. Subjective, secondary data

25. Which type of pain is associated with adverse effects on the sympathetic nervous system?

    A. Acute pain
    B. Chronic pain
    C. Aching pain
    D. Dull pain

26. Select the type of pain that is accurately paired with its characteristics.

    A. Chronic pain: This pain innervates the A delta and C sensory nerves
    B. Acute pain: This pain is associated with ongoing peripheral pain receptor activation
    C. Neuropathic pain: This type of pain is the most difficult to effectively treat
    D. Somatic pain: This type of pain is associated with psychological factors

27. You ask your client where their pain is and the client states, "I really do not know, it is just all over." What type of pain is the client most often affected with?

    A. Somatic pain
    B. Psychogenic pain
    C. Peripheral neuropathic pain
    D. Visceral pain

28. Select the type of pain that is accurately paired with its characteristic(s).

    A. Somatic pain: Vague and not easily located
    B. Neuropathic pain: Can occur with spinal cord injuries
    C. Visceral pain: This pain is described as sharp
    D. Peripheral neuropathic pain: Can occur with spinal cord injuries

29. The process of adjusting the dosage of a medication to achieve the desired effect is referred to as:

    A. Titration
    B. Break through dosage
    C. Rescue dosage
    D. Palliative care

30. Your client's total daily dosage of morphine is 30 mg in 24h and it is given q 4 h using 5 mg of morphine. What would you expect the doctor's order for a rescue dosage to be?

    A. 1 mg of morphine q 1 h
    B. 2 mg of morphine q 1 h
    C. 3 mg of morphine q 1 h
    D. 4 mg of morphine q 1 h

31. Which of the following is considered a unique identifier for the client?

    A. The last four of the client's social security number
    B. The client's room number and nursing unit
    C. The client's middle and surnames
    D. The client's surname and doctor's name

32. Which of the following is an accurate equivalent?

    A. 1 gr = 30 mL
    B. 1 oz. = 60 mg
    C. 1 tsp = 6.5 mL
    D. 1 tbsp. = 15 mL

33. Which is an appropriate expected outcome for a client who is taking an opioid for pain?

    A. The nurse will assess for pain before the administration of the opioid
    B. The nurse will assess for pain before and after the administration of the opioid
    C. The client will express a decrease in their level of pain
    D. The client will maintain adequate circulatory perfusion

34. Which nursing diagnosis is most appropriate for the client who is taking an opioid medication for pain?

    A. At risk for hypertension
    B. At risk for falls
    C. At risk for hallucinations
    D. At risk for elopement

35. Your client has a diastolic blood pressure of 90 and a systolic blood pressure of 197. What is the pulse pressure for this client and what is the most likely cause of this? Select the correct pulse pressure that is paired with the most likely cause of this widening pulse pressure.

    A. 107: Increased intracranial pressure
    B. 90: Cor pulmonale
    C. 197: Increased intracranial pressure
    D. 107: Cor pulmonale

36. How many tablets will you administer to the client with the following order?

    Doctor's order: 6 mg/kg po
    Patient's weight: 230 lbs
    Medication label: 200 mg/tablet

    A. 3
    B. 2
    C. 1
    D. ½

37. How many drops would you administer to an infant with the following order?

    Doctor's order: 5 mg/kg/day in 3 divided doses
    Patient's weight: 4.5 kg
    Medication label: 25 mg/5ml.

    A. 21
    B. 23
    C. 24
    D. 25

38. How many drops per minute will you administer with this intravenous order?

    Doctor's order: 0.9% Na Cl solution at 50 mL per hour and the IV tubing delivers 20 gtts/mL

    A. 14 gtts/min
    B. 15 gtts/min
    C. 16 gtts/min
    D. 17 gtts/min

39. Your client just began to take a new medication and suddenly the client has experienced a seizure. What would you suspect?

    A. A side effect to the medication
    B. Polypharmacy
    C. An adverse effect to the medication
    D. Drug-drug interaction

40. You client is taking an opioid drug and Phenergan in combination to keep the opioid dosage to a minimum. What kind of action is expected with this type of combination?

    A. An inhibiting effect
    B. A potentiating effect
    C. An antagonist effect
    D. An adverse effect

41. The breakdown of a drug, or medication, in the liver is referred to as:

    A. Biotransformation
    B. Distribution
    C. Pharmacokinetics
    D. Absorption

42. Which organization developed the Pain Ladder?

    A. The World Health Organization
    B. The American Nurses Association
    C. The National Board for Certification of Hospice and Palliative Nurses
    D. The American Board for Certification of Hospice and Palliative Nurses

43. A non-pharmacologic intervention for pain is:

    A. Capsaicin cream.
    B. Capsaicin ointment.
    C. Transcutaneous nerve stimulation.
    D. Subcutaneous nerve stimulation.

44. Music therapy is an alternative pain management intervention. What are the four types of music therapy?

    A. Modern, interpretive, re-creative and creative
    B. Receptive, improvisation, re-creative and creative
    C. Expressive, interpretive, creative and expressive
    D. Eclectic, creative, expressive and modern

45. Select the term that is accurately paired with its characteristic or sign and symptom.

    A. Wernicke's aphasia: Expressive aphasia
    B. Broca's aphasia: Receptive aphasia
    C. Broca's aphasia: An inability to comprehend the written word
    D. Wernicke's aphasia: An inability to comprehend the spoken word

46. Which test is used to assess aphasia?

    A. The Rancho Los Amigos Aphasia Test
    B. The Glasgow Aphasia Test
    C. The Boston Diagnostic Aphasia Test
    D. The Billroth Aphasia Test

47. Select the level of consciousness that is accurately paired with its characteristic(s).

    A. Persistent vegetative state: Loss of all motor functioning
    B. Locked In Syndrome: Retained cognitive functioning
    C. A Rancho Los Amigos score of I: Fully alert and conscious
    D. A Rancho Los Amigos score of VIII: Complete unresponsiveness

48. Your client is having non-rhythmic, involuntary muscle jerking of the head and neck muscles. Which nursing diagnosis is most appropriate for your client?

    A. At risk for injury r/t myoclonus
    B. At risk for impaired cardiovascular function r/t hypercalcemia
    C. Poor self-esteem r/t epilepsy
    D. Poor muscular function r/t hypokalemia

49. Select the type of neuropathy that is correctly paired with its characteristic and sign(s).

    A. Symmetric polyneuropathy: Stocking glove type neuropathy; adversely affects the nerve roots from L2 through L4
    B. Autonomic neuropathy: Adversely affects the 4th and 6th cranial nerves; gastroparesis
    C. Radiculopathy: It can involve the cervical and thoracic nerve roots; leg muscle atrophy
    D. Cranial neuropathy: It affects the oculomotor cranial nerve; anisocoria

50. Which type of neuropathy places the client most at risk for foot drop?

    A. Small fiber symmetric neuropathy
    B. Charcot joint neuropathy
    C. Large fiber symmetric neuropathy
    D. Billroth joint neuropathy

51. Your client has a nursing diagnosis of "At risk for seizures r/t brain metastasis." What should you, as the nurse, be aware of?

    A. Cerebral energy and blood flow demands can increase by 50% during a seizure
    B. The tonic phase of a seizure is characterized with alternating periods of muscular relaxation and muscular contraction
    C. The clonic phase of a seizure is characterized with excessive, prolonged muscle contraction
    D. Cerebral energy and blood flow demands can increase by 250% during a seizure

52. Which statement about extrapyramidal symptoms is accurate?

    A. Tardive dyskinesia, which is manifested with involuntary, purposeless movements like lip smacking, is short lived and reversible when the antipsychotic medication is discontinued.
    B. Tardive dyskinesia, which can be permanent, is manifested with involuntary, purposeless movements like lip smacking.
    C. Akathisia is associated with twisting and contractions of the neck area which can be severely painful
    D. Dystonia is associated with severe inner and/or external restlessness, shakiness and jitters.

53. Your client has preserved sensory function and absent motor function below the level of their spinal cord injury. According to the American Spinal Injury Association, their ASIA scale is:

    A. Grade A
    B. Grade B
    C. Grade C
    D. Grade D

54. As you are monitoring the vital signs for your client, you notice that the client's blood pressure is now 180/70. The client's previous blood pressures ran from 144/88 to 168/100. What would you suspect?

    A. A widening pulse pressure and increased intracranial pressure
    B. A pulse pressure of 70 and increased intracranial pressure
    C. A pulse pressure of 110 and a decreased intracranial pressure
    D. A widening pulse pressure and decreased intracranial pressure

55. Select the term that is appropriately paired with its description.

    A. Cushing's reflex: Hypertension, bradycardia, and a narrowing pulse pressure
    B. Decerebrate posturing: Stiff bent arms turned towards the body, clenched fists held on the chest and straight stiff legs
    C. Decorticate posturing: The arms and legs straight out, the toes pointed downward, and the neck and head arched backwards
    D. Cushing's reflex: Hypertension, bradycardia, and a widening pulse pressure

56. One of your clients, a 67 year old female with brain metastasis, is exhibiting decorticate posturing; and another of your clients is a 76 year old male with brain metastasis who is exhibiting decerebrate posturing. Which of these clients is in the most serious condition and why?

    A. The 67 year old female because this client has greater brain damage than the 76 year old male
    B. The 67 year old female because this client is exhibiting Cushing's symptoms
    C. The 76 year old male because this client is exhibiting Cushing's symptoms
    D. The 76 year old male because this client has greater brain damage than the 67 year old female

57. Your client is at the end of life. They have not had any fluids or food for the last 4 days. The client has also not had a bowel movement in the same number of days. What interventional treatment is indicated for this client?

    A. Forcing fluids and a digital disimpaction
    B. No treatment is indicated during these last hours or days of life
    C. A stool softener like docusate or bisacodyl
    D. Increasing both fiber and fluids

58. Which is the most frequent cause of hiccups?

    A. Gastric distension
    B. Hepatic tumors
    C. Brain stem lesions
    D. Corticosteroids

59. Crede massage is used to promote:

    A. Urination
    B. Relaxation
    C. Sleep
    D. Defecation

60. Urinary retention is defined as:

    A. 35% or more of residual after voiding.
    B. 45% or more of residual after voiding.
    C. More than 100 ml of residual.
    D. More than 200 ml of residual.

61. "At risk for disuse syndrome" is an appropriate nursing diagnosis for a client who is affected with:

    A. Failure to thrive
    B. Deconditioning
    C. Nephritis
    D. Diabetic ketoacidosis

62. As you are dangling the client at the edge of the bed, the client's vital signs change and the client is dizzy, pale and nauseated. What is this client most likely affected with?

    A. Cardiac tamponade
    B. Pleural effusion
    C. Left sided heart failure
    D. Activity intolerance

63. Fear and anxiety are similar; however, they are also different. One difference between fear and anxiety is that fear is:

    A. Typically related to a future threat
    B. Typically related to a current threat
    C. Only results from imagined threats
    D. Only results from real threats

64. When all possible causes of agitation and restlessness have been eliminated, the physician may prescribe medications, such as:

    A. Corticosteroids and antidepressants
    B. Corticosteroids and anticonvulsants
    C. Antianxiety and antipsychotics
    D. Antidepressants and anticonvulsants

65. Which fact about distress is accurate?

    A. Distress is not influenced by the stage or site of a disease
    B. Distress occurs only in clients with life-threatening illnesses
    C. Distress only occurs at the end of life
    D. Distress is a common occurrence throughout the illness continuum

66. Select the psychological defense mechanism that is correctly paired with its description.

    A. Reaction formation: The client acts out in a manner that is the same of what their true feelings are
    B. Sublimation: A normal sexual or aggressive urge is replaced with a socially unacceptable sexual or aggressive urge
    C. Undoing: Allows the client to feel as though they have made up for, and atoned, for wrong doing
    D. Compensation: Hostility is moved from one person or object to another

67. Your HIV/AIDS client is blaming others for their disease. Which psychological defense mechanism is this client employing?

    A. Displacement
    B. Regression
    C. Sublimation
    D. Projection

68. Your client has terminal cancer and the client's daughter has expressed extreme sorrow about their mother and their mother's impending death. What type of loss is this daughter most likely experiencing?

    A. Perceived loss
    B. Anticipatory loss
    C. Actual loss
    D. Profound loss

69. Which theorist has shock, awareness of the loss, conservation, healing and renewal as the phases of bereavement?

    A. Sander
    B. Kubler-Ross
    C. Engel
    D. Piaget

70. The primary purpose of feeling guilty is to:

    A. Punish the person for a wrongdoing
    B. Change behaviors
    C. Get attention away from a negative behavior
    D. Allow for time to rest

71. Select the level of awareness that is correctly paired with its description.

    A. Closed awareness: An unawareness of impending death and terminal illness
    B. Mutual pretense: When the client and their loved ones openly discuss the client's condition
    C. Mutual pretense: When the caregiver openly explains to only the client about their impending death
    D. Open awareness: When the client is aware of their condition and impending death, but their loved ones do not

72. Select the sleep disturbance that is accurately paired with its sign, symptom or complication.

    A. Insomnia: Inability to remain asleep, but able to fall asleep
    B. Insomnia: Inability to fall asleep, but able to remain asleep
    C. Hypersomnia: The client is unable to stay awake in the daytime even after a good night sleep
    D. Sleep apnea: Excessive bouts of uncontrollable sleep attacks throughout the daytime

73. Under what circumstance does confidentiality have to be legally violated?

    A. When the client is infected with a terminal disease
    B. When the client expresses thoughts of suicide
    C. When the client is unable to speak
    D. When the client is unable to see

74. Which underlying condition is the most frequent cause of sexual dysfunction among cancer clients?

    A. The loss of sexual desire
    B. Depression
    C. Anxiety
    D. Body image alterations

75. Your client at the end of life is severely anorexic. Which of the following is this client most prone to?

    A. Depression
    B. Loss of purpose
    C. Cachexia
    D. Hopelessness

76. Your client has dry mouth and excessive thirst, what disorder are they most likely to have?

    A. Dehydration
    B. Diabetic ketoacidosis
    C. Diabetes insipidus
    D. Diabetes mellitus

77. Which nursing diagnosis is the most appropriate for the client with dry mouth and excessive thirst?

    A. Hallucinations r/t depression
    B. Shortness of breath r/t anxiety
    C. Confusion r/t dehydration
    D. Confusion r/t anxiety

78. Which of the following is an electrolyte with a negative charge?

    A. Chloride
    B. Potassium
    C. Sodium
    D. Calcium

79. What is the normal blood calcium level?

    A. 2.4 - 4.1 mg/dL
    B. 1.7-2.2 mg/dL
    C. 96-106 milliequivalents (mEq) per liter
    D. 8.5-10.6 mg/dL

80. What is the normal blood phosphorus level?.

    A. 2.4-4.1 mg/dL
    B. 1.7-2.2 mg/dL
    C. 96-106 milliequivalents (mEq) per liter
    D. 8.5-10.6 mg/dL

81. What is the normal blood potassium level?

    A. 1.7-2.2 mg/dL
    B. 3.7-5.2 mEq/L
    C. 96-106 milliequivalents (mEq) per liter
    D. 8.5-10.6 mg/dL

82. What disorder occurs as a result of either not consuming or absorbing enough magnesium or excreting too much magnesium?

    A. Hypermagnesemia
    B. Hypomagnesemia
    C. Hypermagnesium
    D. Hypomagnesium

83. MODY occurs as the result of:

    A. Hyperthyroidism
    B. Hypothyroidism
    C. A single gene mutation
    D. Multiple gene mutations

84. Your client has a mutation in the gene that encodes a protein called glucokinase. What is this client most likely affected with?

    A. Diabetes ketoacidosis
    B. Maturity-onset diabetes (MODY)
    C. Diabetes insipidus
    D. Diabetes mellitus

85. The first three phases of grieving in correct sequential order, according to Engel's theory include:

    A. Shock and disbelief, developing awareness and restitution
    B. Developing awareness, shock and renewal
    C. Developing awareness, shock and restitution
    D. Shock, awareness of the loss and conservation and withdrawal

86. Whose theory of grieving includes the unique phase of bargaining?

    A. Engel's
    B. Sander's
    C. Maslow's
    D. Kubler Ross's

87. What leads to three of the most commonly occurring complications of diabetes, namely, retinopathy, nephropathy and neuropathy?

    A. Cardiac arrest
    B. Arterial flutter
    C. Microvascular damage
    D. Macrovascular damage

88. Which is the most commonly occurring form of diabetic neuropathy?

    A. Radiculopathy
    B. Cranial neuropathy
    C. Symmetric polyneuropathy
    D. Autonomic neuropathy

89. What is the single most effective way to prevent nosocomial infections in our healthcare facilities?

    A. Changing open wound dressings
    B. Disinfection
    C. Sterilization
    D. Hand washing

90. Which term describes a decrease in cells that are responsible for carrying oxygen, providing immunity, and normal blood clotting cells?

    A. Myelosuppression
    B. Rhabdomyolysis
    C. Hypokalemia
    D. Hyperkalemia

91. Select the term that is correctly paired with its description.

    A. Anemia: An increase in the oxygen carrying red blood cells
    B. Neutropenia: A decrease in the number of white blood cells, or neutrophils
    C. Thrombocytopenia: An increase in the number of platelets in the blood
    D. Disseminated intravascular coagulation: Too much sodium in the blood

92. Your client has just completed a course of chemotherapy and is now affected with nosebleeds, gum bleeding, and petechia. Which disorder would you suspect?

    A. Thrombocytopenia
    B. Anemia
    C. Neutropenia
    D. Transplant rejection

93. Compression sleeves are used for the treatment of:

    A. Lymphedema.
    B. Thrombocytopenia.
    C. Anemia.
    D. Neutropenia.

94. Which is an appropriate expected outcome for a client who is taking an opioid for pain?

    A. The client will maintain adequate oxygenation
    B. The client will express a decrease in their pain
    C. The nurse will assess for pain before the administration of the opioid
    D. The nurse will assess for pain before and after the administration of the opioid

95. Select the term that is correctly paired with its description.

    A. Lymphedema: Abnormal swelling of the arm(s) and/or leg(s) that results from a blockage in the lymphatic system
    B. Myelosuppression: A decrease in the oxygen carrying red blood cells
    C. Anemia: A decrease in cells responsible for carrying oxygen, providing immunity, and normal blood clotting
    D. Disseminated intravascular coagulation: High levels of potassium in the blood

96. The third sequential step of the evaluation process is:

    A. Data collection relating to the expected outcome
    B. Data analysis and comparison of the data to the outcomes
    C. Relating the interventions to the expected outcomes
    D. Concluding about the client's problem status

97. Which fact about Medicare hospice benefits is accurate?

    A. Medicare hospice benefits cover an unlimited number of 60 day benefit periods as long as the client continues to meet the eligibility criteria under Medicare Part A benefits
    B. Medicare hospice benefits do not cover 90 day benefit periods at any time
    C. It is not necessary to report changes in a client's condition or death until the Medicare hospice quarterly update is due
    D. Medicare hospice benefits are only available for clients who are in a hospice facility not at home hospice care

98. Which Medicare part reimburses for immunosuppressive drugs for organ transplant clients?

    A. Part A
    B. Part B
    C. Part C
    D. Part D

99. Your hospice client is returning home and is in need of some things like a walker and a bedside commode. How are items like this reimbursed for?

    A. Part A
    B. Part B
    C. Part C
    D. Part D

100. Your client has an ordered narcotic analgesic q 4 h. At 10 am. You remove the medication from the locked cabinet and administer the medication to the client. When should you document this medication?

    A. Immediately after removing it from the locked cabinet and immediately after administering it
    B. Immediately after the client has taken the medication
    C. Its removal from the locked cabinet and its administration should be documented just before administration
    D. None of the above is true

101. Which of the following factors does not affect the communication process during the nurse-client relationship?

    A. Time of day
    B. Perceptions
    C. Emotions
    D. Pain

102. Which is a barrier to communication?

    A. Challenging the client's thoughts
    B. Silence during conversation
    C. Probing in order to get more insight into the client's perspectives
    D. Paraphrasing the client's statements

103. Which therapeutic communication technique can be both therapeutic as well as nontherapeutic in the nurse-client relationship?

    A. Silence
    B. Paraphrasing
    C. Providing leads
    D. Listening

104. The five phases of life review include:

   A. Responsibility, forgiveness, acceptance, realization, and gratitude.
   B. Expression, responsibility, forgiveness, acceptance, and gratitude.
   C. Reaction, expression, realization, forgiveness, and acceptance.
   D. Reaction, realization, acceptance, forgiveness, and gratitude.

105. Which statement about the role of the nurse in caregiver support is true?

   A. Caregivers do not have to be given support by the nurse or any other member of the team
   B. Caregiver support facilitates the caregiver's confidence and competence
   C. Caregiver support decreases the costs of healthcare
   D. Caregiver support allows for longer hospitalization time

106. Your client is able to perform some functional self-care activities, but not all. Which assessment should the hospice and palliative care nurse perform in order to determine the reason for this partly compensatory nursing system, according to Orem's theory?

   A. The client's cultural background
   B. The client's musculoskeletal functioning
   C. The client's level of cognition
   D. All of the above

107. Select the client with the type of nursing system, according to Dorothea Orem's Self-Care theory.

   A. A 54 year old client in a coma: Wholly compensatory nursing system
   B. An infant: Supportive nursing system
   C. A 76 year old client who is able to perform all self-care independently: Supportive-educative nursing system
   D. A 23 year old client with leukemia who needs some assistance with personal hygiene: Wholly compensatory nursing system

108. You are teaching your client about the proper care of a new colostomy. What domain of learning are you teaching?

   A. Pedagogy
   B. Cognitive
   C. Affective
   D. Psychomotor

109. An expected outcome for an educational activity relating to the proper use of a TENS machine is:

   A. The nurse will demonstrate the proper use of a TENS machine.
   B. The nurse will discuss the importance of a TENS machine.
   C. The client will demonstrate the proper use of a TENS machine.
   D. The client will discuss the importance of a TENS machine.

110. Culture affects which aspects of the teaching/learning process?

   A. Communication and terminology use
   B. Tolerance for low lighting and communication
   C. The ambient temperature of the room and stress levels
   D. Teaching strategies and terminology use

111. Which is a motivator?

   A. High stress
   B. No stress
   C. Moderate stress
   D. Low stress

112. Your client is not able to fully understand information enough to be able to use it to make appropriate health care decisions. Which barrier to learning does this client most likely have?

   A. Health illiteracy
   B. Lack of motivation
   C. A cognitive impairment
   D. High level stress

113. One of the most effective ways to motivate caregiver learners is to:

   A. Listen and hear all of the client's concerns and fears.
   B. Have the client actively participate in all phases of the teaching.
   C. Have the caregiver actively participate in all phases of the teaching.
   D. Provide a quiet and comfortable environment without distractions.

114. Encouraging the learner to reflect on readings, contemplate applications and summarize material rather than the memorizing facts is an effective strategy for a client with which type of learning style or preference?

    A. Active learning
    B. Visual learning
    C. Reflective learning
    D. Intuitive learning

115. Which learning style characterizes learners who prefer detail oriented learning and practical, real world oriented learning rather than abstraction?

    A. Sensing learners
    B. Reflective learners
    C. Intuitive learners
    D. Verbal learners

116. Which phase of the decision making process is most prone to errors?

    A. Ranking and weighing criteria
    B. Deciding on the best alternative
    C. Problem definition
    D. Implementing the course of action

117. Which regulatory body enforces regulations relating to biohazardous waste and sharps disposal in the community?

    A. U.S. Environmental Protection Agency
    B. Occupational Safety and Health Administration
    C. Centers for Disease Control
    D. Centers for Medicare and Medicaid Services

118. Which term is most closely associated with medical necessity?

    A. Reimbursement
    B. Ethics
    C. Qui Tam
    D. Respondeat Superior

119. Hospice and palliative care nurses perform values histories. What is the primary purpose of a values history?

   A. To guide unanticipated decision making when the client is no longer able to perform this function
   B. To determine the client's and significant others' priorities in terms of importance
   C. To determine the client's and significant others' priorities in terms of physical and spiritual needs
   D. To guide decision making in terms of the client's advance directives while they are competent to do so

120. Successful delegation is most dependent on:

   A. The legal and appropriate matching of client needs with staff competencies
   B. The leadership and conflict resolution skills of the person who is delegating
   C. The preferences of the clients, significant others and staff members
   D. Specificity of the delegated assignments and follow up supervision

121. Which four levels of hospice care are reimbursed, as based on the level of care the agencies provide?

   A. Respite care, general inpatient care, intensive care, and clinical care
   B. Respite care up to 6 days, home care, general inpatient care, and clinical care
   C. Routine home care, continuous home care, respite care, and general inpatient care
   D. Respite care, home care, intensive care, and clinical care

122. During which phase of group process does conflict among group members begin?

   A. The storming phase
   B. The forming phase
   C. The norming phase
   D. Conflict should never occur

123. Select the phase of team building that is correctly paired with its description.

   A. Forming: the members of the new group are asked a series of questions by the already existing members
   B. Storming: Phase when conflicts arise
   C. Norming: The new members get to know each other and the purpose of the group
   D. Performing: The group establishes its expectations

124. Which type of decision making, within the nurse-client relationship, is the most beneficial to the client?

   A. Shared decision making because the autonomous client gets the professional support of the nurse
   B. Patient sovereignty decision making because it includes the client
   C. Paternalistic decision making because the nurse, as the expert, insures that the client makes the correct decision
   D. Caring decision making, because the client and their loved ones are included

125. Volunteers:

   A. Need an orientation and policies and procedures to insure their competency.
   B. Do not need an orientation because they are not paid as hospital staff.
   C. Have minimal and insignificant contributions to end of life care.
   D. Are not suited for supportive care at the end of life for hospice clients.

126. The National Hospice and Palliative Care Organization's standard of practice that encourages the universal availability of palliative and hospice care services is referred to as:

   A. Accessibility to insure that the needs of the underserved are met
   B. Referral in order to insure the appropriate level of care as based on need
   C. Equality in order to insure that all clients are treated at the same level of care
   D. Universality of human physical and emotional needs at the end of life

127. Select the ethical term that is correctly and accurately paired with its description.

   A. Beneficence: "Do not harm", as in the Hippocratic Oath
   B. Justice: Truthfulness and honesty
   C. Nonmaleficence: "Do not harm", as in the Hippocratic Oath
   D. Fidelity: Fairness and equality

128. Which fact about a bereavement program is accurate?

   A. Bereavement services are recognized as a core component of the palliative care program
   B. Bereavement services and follow-up are made available to the family for a maximum of 6 months
   C. Bereavement services and follow-up are usually only needed when the bereaved spouse is very young
   D. Bereavement service are an accessory, rather than core, component of the palliative care program

129. What is the name of the process used to dig down to the deepest, real reasons why mistakes and errors have occurred?

   A. Peer review
   B. Root cause analysis
   C. Variance tracking
   D. Benchmarking

130. Which term best describes the nurse's application of research findings into practice?

   A. Benchmarking practice
   B. Evidence based practice
   C. Professional decision making
   D. Critical thinking practice

131. What is hypokalemia?

   A. High levels of phosphorus in the blood
   B. Low levels of phosphorus in the blood
   C. High levels of potassium in the blood
   D. Low levels of potassium in the blood

132. Many end of life choices revolve around which issue?

   A. Critical care issues
   B. Quality of life issues
   C. Intensive care issues
   D. Nurse's issues

133. If a client has been administered a sedative, and they in turn react with agitation rather than sedation, this is known as:

   A. A cumulative effect
   B. A therapeutic effect
   C. An idiosyncratic effect
   D. A potentiating effect

134. If a controlled substance is wasted, entirely or partially, the waste must be witnessed by:

   A. The wasting nurse and the client.
   B. Two nurses in addition to the wasting nurse.
   C. The wasting nurse alone.
   D. The wasting nurse and another nurse.

135. Conflicts arise when there are disparate:

    A. Opinions, values, beliefs and attitudes
    B. Opinions, causes, religions and attitudes
    C. Causes, religions, beliefs and values
    D. Causes, beliefs, values and attitudes

136. The best way to resolve conflicts is by:

    A. Trying to convince others to agree with you
    B. Communication and collaboration
    C. Coercion
    D. Taking a vote or flipping a coin

137. Which of the following medications is used to treat mild to moderate pain?

    A. Hydromorphone
    B. Methadone
    C. Morphine
    D. Codeine

138. Which of the following medications is only available in combination with other ingredients?

    A. Fentanyl
    B. Hydrocodone
    C. Codeine
    D. Morphine

139. Which of the following medications is classified as an opioid?

    A. Fentanyl
    B. Budesonide
    C. Topiramate
    D. Beclomethasone

140. Which of the following medications is classified as a NSAID?

    A. Beclomethasone
    B. Budesonide
    C. Etodolac
    D. Topiramate

141. Which is used for the short-term management of moderately severe acute pain that otherwise could require narcotics?

   A. Diflunisal
   B. Meclofenamate
   C. Mefenamic acid
   D. Ketorolac

142. Which of the following medications is classified as a corticosteroid?

   A. Diclofenac
   B. Piroxicam
   C. Triamcinolone
   D. Levetiracetam

143. Which of the following corticosteroids is given both orally and with injection?

   A. Methylprednisolone
   B. Flurbiprofen
   C. Celecoxib
   D. Phenytoin

144. Which of the following medications is classified as an anticonvulsant?

   A. Triamcinolone
   B. Phenytoin
   C. Mometasone
   D. Ketoprofen

145. Which of the following anticonvulsants is used to treat chronic low back pain, cancer pain and neuropathic pain?

   A. Levetiracetam
   B. Carbamazepine
   C. Topiramate
   D. Pregabalin

146. Which of the following medications is a tricyclic antidepressant?

   A. Maprotiline
   B. Zonisamide
   C. Oxycarbazepine
   D. Piroxicam

147. Which of the following tricyclic antidepressants is available in an oral capsule, concentrate and a topical?

   A. Nortriptyline
   B. Doxepin
   C. Trazodone
   D. Despramine

148. Which of the following medications is indicated for a client with low back pain?

   A. Oxycarbazepine
   B. Valproic acid
   C. Trazodone
   D. Maprotiline

149. Which of the following is NOT a symptom of dysphagia?

   A. Pain in the extremities
   B. Frequent heartburn
   C. Hoarseness
   D. Drooling

150. Which of the following opioids has a usual dosage of 30mg q 1-6h?

   A. Hydrocodone
   B. Codeine
   C. Hydromorphone
   D. Fentanyl

ANSWER KEY

1. Answer: B
2. Answer: A
3. Answer: D
4. Answer: D
5. Answer: B
6. Answer: C
7. Answer: A
8. Answer: C
9. Answer: B
10. Answer: D
11. Answer: A
12. Answer: C
13. Answer: C
14. Answer: B
15. Answer: A
16. Answer: A
17. Answer: A
18. Answer: C
19. Answer: D
20. Answer: D
21. Answer: C
22. Answer: A
23. Answer: C
24. Answer: A
25. Answer: A
26. Answer: C
27. Answer: D
28. Answer: B
29. Answer: A
30. Answer: C
31. Answer: A
32. Answer: D
33. Answer: C
34. Answer: B
35. Answer: A
36. Answer: A
37. Answer: B
38. Answer: D
39. Answer: C
40. Answer: B
41. Answer: D
42. Answer: A
43. Answer: C

44. Answer: B
45. Answer: D
46. Answer: C
47. Answer: B
48. Answer: A
49. Answer: D
50. Answer: C
51. Answer: D
52. Answer: B
53. Answer: B
54. Answer: A
55. Answer: D
56. Answer: D
57. Answer: B
58. Answer: A
59. Answer: A
60. Answer: D
61. Answer: B
62. Answer: D
63. Answer: B
64. Answer: C
65. Answer: D
66. Answer: C
67. Answer: D
68. Answer: B
69. Answer: A
70. Answer: B
71. Answer: A
72. Answer: C
73. Answer: B
74. Answer: A
75. Answer: C
76. Answer: A
77. Answer: C
78. Answer: A
79. Answer: D
80. Answer: A
81. Answer: B
82. Answer: B
83. Answer: C
84. Answer: B
85. Answer: A
86. Answer: D
87. Answer: C
88. Answer: C

89. Answer: D
90. Answer: A
91. Answer: B
92. Answer: A
93. Answer: A
94. Answer: B
95. Answer: A
96. Answer: C
97. Answer: A
98. Answer: B
99. Answer: B
100. Answer: A
101. Answer: A
102. Answer: A
103. Answer: A
104. Answer: B
105. Answer: B
106. Answer: D
107. Answer: A
108. Answer: D
109. Answer: C
110. Answer: A
111. Answer: C
112. Answer: A
113. Answer: C
114. Answer: C
115. Answer: A
116. Answer: C
117. Answer: A
118. Answer: A
119. Answer: A
120. Answer: A
121. Answer: C
122. Answer: A
123. Answer: B
124. Answer: A
125. Answer: A
126. Answer: A
127. Answer: C
128. Answer: A
129. Answer: B
130. Answer: B
131. Answer: C
132. Answer: B
133. Answer: C

134. Answer: D
135. Answer: A
136. Answer: B
137. Answer: D
138. Answer: B
139. Answer: A
140. Answer: C
141. Answer: D
142. Answer: C
143. Answer: A
144. Answer: B
145. Answer: D
146. Answer: A
147. Answer: B
148. Answer: D
149. Answer: A
150. Answer: B

Exclusive Trivium Test Tips

Here at Trivium Test Prep, we strive to offer you the exemplary test tools that help you pass your exam the first time. This book includes an overview of important concepts, example questions throughout the text, and practice test questions. But we know that learning how to successfully take a test can be just as important as learning the content being tested. In addition to excelling on the CHPN, we want to give you the solutions you need to be successful every time you take a test. Our study strategies, preparation pointers, and test tips will help you succeed as you take the CHPN and any test in the future!

Study Strategies

1. Spread out your studying. By taking the time to study a little bit every day, you strengthen your understanding of the testing material, so it's easier to recall that information on the day of the test. Our study guides make this easy by breaking up the concepts into sections with example practice questions, so you can test your knowledge as you read.
2. Create a study calendar. The sections of our book make it easy to review and practice with example questions on a schedule. Decide to read a specific number of pages or complete a number of practice questions every day. Breaking up all of the information in this way can make studying less overwhelming and more manageable.
3. Set measurable goals and motivational rewards. Follow your study calendar and reward yourself for completing reading, example questions, and practice problems and tests. You could take yourself out after a productive week of studying or watch a favorite show after reading a chapter. Treating yourself to rewards is a great way to stay motivated.
4. Use your current knowledge to understand new, unfamiliar concepts. When you learn something new, think about how it relates to something you know really well. Making connections between new ideas and your existing understanding can simplify the learning process and make the new information easier to remember.
5. Make learning interesting! If one aspect of a topic is interesting to you, it can make an entire concept easier to remember. Stay engaged and think about how concepts covered on the exam can affect the things you're interested in. The sidebars throughout the text offer additional information that could make ideas easier to recall.
6. Find a study environment that works for you. For some people, absolute silence in a library results in the most effective study session, while others need the background noise of a coffee shop to fuel productive studying. There are many websites that generate white noise and recreate the sounds of different environments for studying. Figure out what distracts you and what engages you and plan accordingly.
7. Take practice tests in an environment that reflects the exam setting. While it's important to be as comfortable as possible when you study, practicing taking the test exactly as you'll take it on test day will make you more prepared for the actual exam. If your test starts on a Saturday morning, take your practice test on a Saturday morning. If you have access, try to

find an empty classroom that has desks like the desks at testing center. The more closely you can mimic the testing center, the more prepared you'll feel on test day.
8. Study hard for the test in the days before the exam, but take it easy the night before and do something relaxing rather than studying and cramming. This will help decrease anxiety, allow you to get a better night's sleep, and be more mentally fresh during the big exam. Watch a light-hearted movie, read a favorite book, or take a walk, for example.

Preparation Pointers

1. Preparation is key! Don't wait until the day of your exam to gather your pencils, calculator, identification materials, or admission tickets. Check the requirements of the exam as soon as possible. Some tests require materials that may take more time to obtain, such as a passport-style photo, so be sure that you have plenty of time to collect everything. The night before the exam, lay out everything you'll need, so it's all ready to go on test day! We recommend at least two forms of ID, your admission ticket or confirmation, pencils, a high protein, compact snack, bottled water, and any necessary medications. Some testing centers will require you to put all of your supplies in a clear plastic bag. If you're prepared, you will be less stressed the morning of, and less likely to forget anything important.
2. If you're taking a pencil-and-paper exam, test your erasers on paper. Some erasers leave big, dark stains on paper instead of rubbing out pencil marks. Make sure your erasers work for you and the pencils you plan to use.
3. Make sure you give yourself your usual amount of sleep, preferably at least 7 – 8 hours. You may find you need even more sleep. Pay attention to how much you sleep in the days before the exam, and how many hours it takes for you to feel refreshed. This will allow you to be as sharp as possible during the test and make fewer simple mistakes.
4. Make sure to make transportation arrangements ahead of time, and have a backup plan in case your ride falls through. You don't want to be stressing about how you're going to get to the testing center the morning of the exam.
5. Many testing locations keep their air conditioners on high. You want to remember to bring a sweater or jacket in case the test center is too cold, as you never know how hot or cold the testing location could be. Remember, while you can always adjust for heat by removing layers, if you're cold, you're cold.

Test Tips

1. Go with your gut when choosing an answer. Statistically, the answer that comes to mind first is often the right one. This is assuming you studied the material, of course, which we hope you have done if you've read through one of our books!
2. For true or false questions: if you genuinely don't know the answer, mark it true. In most tests, there are typically more true answers than false answers.
3. For multiple-choice questions, read ALL the answer choices before marking an answer, even if you think you know the answer when you come across it. You may find your original "right" answer isn't necessarily the best option.

4. Look for key words: in multiple choice exams, particularly those that require you to read through a text, the questions typically contain key words. These key words can help the test taker choose the correct answer or confuse you if you don't recognize them. Common keywords are: *most*, *during*, *after*, *initially*, and *first*. Be sure you identify them before you read the available answers. Identifying the key words makes a huge difference in your chances of passing the test.
5. Narrow answers down by using the process of elimination: after you understand the question, read each answer. If you don't know the answer right away, use the process of elimination to narrow down the answer choices. It is easy to identify at least one answer that isn't correct. Continue to narrow down the choices before choosing the answer you believe best fits the question. By following this process, you increase your chances of selecting the correct answer.
6. Don't worry if others finish before or after you. Go at your own pace, and focus on the test in front of you.
7. Relax. With our help, we know you'll be ready to conquer the CHPN. You've studied and worked hard!

Keep in mind that every individual takes tests differently, so strategies that might work for you may not work for someone else. You know yourself best and are the best person to determine which of these tips and strategies will benefit your studying and test taking. Best of luck as you study, test, and work toward your future!

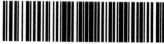

Made in the USA
Middletown, DE
09 January 2017